AF430624

Applied Statistics with Applications in Epidemiological Studies

Applied Statistics with Applications in Epidemiological Studies

Panchaksharappa Gowda D.H.

Asst. Professor, JSS College of Pharmacy,

Sri Shivarathreeshwara Nagar, Mysuru.

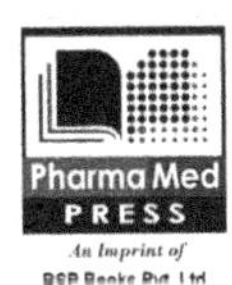

PharmaMed Press

An imprint of BSP Books Pvt. Ltd.

4-4-309/316, Giriraj Lane,

Sultan Bazar, Hyderabad - 500 095.

Published by

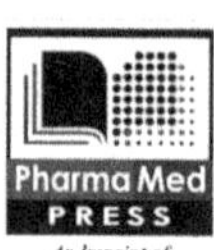

PharmaMed Press

An imprint of BSP Books Pvt. Ltd.

4-4-309/316, Giriraj Lane, Sultan Bazar, Hyderabad - 500 095.

Phone: 040-23445688; Fax: 91+40-23445611

E-mail: info@pharmamedpress.net

www.bspbooks.net/www.pharmamedpress.net

ISBN: 978-93-91910-04-4

PREFACE

This book mainly explains the importance of Biostatistics and its application in epidemiological research or study. I have written this book to help researchers and Biostatisticians understand the application of Biostatistics to analyze the data of epidemiological study by designing mathematical models. This book has explained how to design mathematical models like logistic regression (multiple and straightforward) models. However, most of the data collected from the epidemiological investigations are taken from earlier publications—the references used as a helping tool to write this book are extensively listed in the book.

The primary purpose is to make the distinct and complementary roles of Epidemiology and Biostatistics to Public health.

This book mainly presents the concepts in a clear, concise and accurate manner. The mathematical ratios, mathematical equations and kinetics models considered primary tools to carry out epidemiological study are explained. The book highlights the importance of Probability theory and its application in the computation of proportional values whenever both exposure (independent) variables and outcome events (dependent variable) are considered binary values in designing the simple regression and logistic regression model to analyze the experimental data.

This book would be handy for M.Sc Medical statistics students, researcher scholars in their epidemiological research.

-Author

CONTENTS

CHAPTER 1

Introduction to Health and Epidemiology

Health

Before we conduct epidemiological studies, it is necessary to understand the meaning and definition of health. The widely accepted definition of health as stated by the World Health Organization (1948) in the preamble to its constitution is "Health is a state of complete Physical, Mental and Social well-being and not merely an absence of disease or infirmity".

In the recent years this statement has shown its interest to include the ability to lead a socially and economically productive life. But the WHO definition of health has been criticized as being too broad. One group or many argue that health cannot be defined as "State" at all, but it must be seen as a process of continuous adjustment to the changing demands of living and of the changing means, we give to the life. It is a dynamic concept, it helps people in the society to live well, work well and enjoy life, which every human being expects in life. Some consider it is an irrelevant definition for everyday demands, as nobody qualifies as healthy when the perfect biological, psychological and social aspects are considered. If we accept the WHO definition of health, we cannot find healthy people, as everybody will be sick for one reason or the other.

But this definition only symbolizes the aspirations of people and represents an overall objective or goal towards which our nation and world should strive. Therefore the WHO definition of health can be taken as an idealistic goal than a realistic proposition. According to that definition, it may exist in few individuals, rather than everyone all the time.

In addition to the above mentioned three dimension, WHO can explore the possibility of including the spiritual dimension. According to the vision of health profession "Health for all by 2020", we the people of this world, should focus on spiritual dimension. The public should be aware of what is spirituality in true sense, its impact and benefits by adopting this dimension.

In true sense the spiritual dimension is not going to explain about any religion, but it mainly directs the people of the world on how one should live and work with their true nature. In reality the true nature in the society is, everyone should work in a state of nobody and content.

In general, spiritual dimension is striving to explain and reach each individual by explaining what is life and what is the purpose of life. This spirituality explains the factors which can be considered as root cause for few diseases. The very meaning and purpose of life is to be happy for no reason. This can be achieved, when the people of a particular profession work in a state of nobody and work with content.

The spiritual dimension is described and is interpreted as the need for, meaning, purpose and fulfillment of life. It is important to gain overall sense of health, well-being and quality of life (referred to as the health potential).

The important spiritual values are the truth, righteousness, peace, love and non-violence. These spiritual values are also human values and are fundamental roots of a healthy, vibrant and viable work career.

The spiritual dimension is the tangible "Something" that transcends physiology and psychology. It will transfer from somebody to nobody state.

Determinants of Health

The term 'determinants of health' refer to those factors that have a significant influence, whether positive or negative, on health. The term should not imply a cause–effect relationship between a risk factor and a health status. Health is the result of multiple factors including the genetic, biological, and lifestyle factors related to the individual and the factors relating to the structure of society and its policies.

Epidemiology

Epidemiology is the basic science of preventive and social medicine. It has evolved rapidly during the past decades. In general epidemiology can be defined as the study of distribution and determinants of disease in human population. The first known epidemiologist, also named as father of medicine who has given a major contribution to epidemiology is the Greek Physician Hippocrates (460-377 BCE). Hippocrates has explained how a particular disease is related to time, season, place and environment of the place where they are living. The important factors of the environment are water and change in season. Some excellent epidemiologic studies were conducted before 20th century, but design and evaluation of epidemiological studies began only in the second half of the 20th century. This epidemiology began with Adam and Eve, both trying to investigate the qualities of the "Forbidden Fruit". The word Epidemiology is derived from the word Epidemic (Epi = Among; demos = People; logos = Study). Many of the epidemiological studies were initiated on large scale, in the year 1940. The public health problems were established through observed or measured phenomena in the population of interest. For example, the community-intervention trail of fluoride supplementation in water that was started during the year 1940 gave the solution to prevent dental caries. Later in 1949, the Framingham heart study, was initiated and focused on several long-term follow-up studies of cardiovascular disease, that has contributed to understand the causes of enormous public health problems.

Its ramifications covers not only study of distributions and causation (and thereby Preventive), but also health and health-related events occurring in human populations. Presently the medical sciences in epidemiology has given rise to newer off-shoots such as infectious disease epidemiology, clinical epidemiology, cancer epidemiology, occupational epidemiology, neuro epidemiology, corona study etc.

These studies have added substantially to the advancement of medical knowledge is indisputable. The main concern of the society was the investigation and prevention of infectious diseases. It has been firmly established in medical education and research. Epidemiology identifies the distribution of diseases, factors which are the sources and cause, and methods for their control of diseases which are caused by different factors. This requires an understanding of how political, social and some scientific factors which intersect to increase the risk of the disease, which makes epidemiology a unique science.

In general we can say that epidemiology is a science which has multidisciplinary approach to the study of human health and disease. It applies various techniques of systematic observation, and the formulation, testing, and modification of hypotheses. Generally epidemiology is a highly complex science as it has to focus on different types of variables which are associated with human diseases, such as pathogens, human social or travel dynamics, and the environment etc.

The community and public health medicine very often uses the concept and tools of epidemiology. Epidemiologists study the mechanism, how and why diseases and health related problems arise and how these diseases are distributed among population. The epidemiologist and public professional are interested in studying, why and what are the risk factors for getting the disease and why some members of the population, are free from the disease.

Epidemiology study mainly focuses on the factors, which are associated with induction, promotion and expression of a disease. These risk factors can also be called as explanatory variables, predictor, covariates, independent variables and exposure variables.

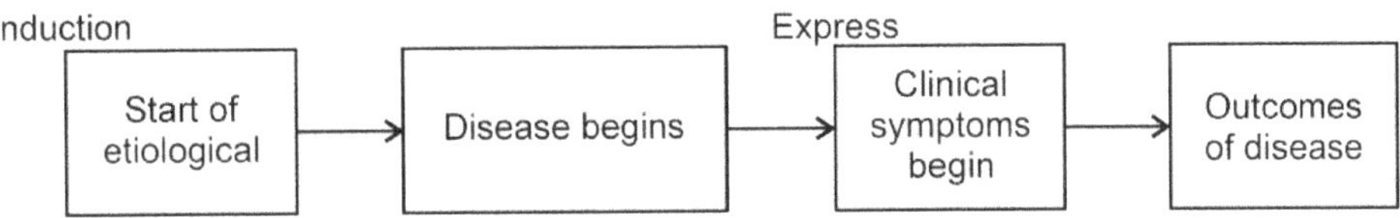

Flow chart of Disease Evolution

In addition to these factors, there are certain factors associated, during induction, promotion and expression which are different from the above factors.

For example, malnutrition is a factor which is associated during induction and promotion stages.

But in disease like coronary heart disease CHD, we can consider three other factors, which are associated with the above factors like dietary factors associated with induction, high blood pressure with promotion, and age and sex with expression.

Disease intervention is of course a very important mechanism to prevent the development of diseases in the entire universe or population. But the intervention strategies vary depending on whether the purpose is to prevent induction, promotion or expression. Public health intervention mainly focus on induction and expression, where as clinical trial or treatment is designed with an intension to alter the expression or the final stage of a disease.

But in epidemiological study, three major components, on which one has to focus   are (i) Studies of disease frequency (ii) Studies of distribution and iii) studies of determinants.

These three components spread an important message to the public health.

Aims of Epidemiology:

The three main aims of epidemiology are listed below

(i)   To find out the distribution and size of the disease problem in the world

(ii) To find the aetiological factors, which are considered as root cause for disease

(iii) To collect and provide the data which is very much required for planning, implementation and evaluation of data, which is required by the authority, who is going do service for the prevention, control and for treating the disease

The ultimate aim of epidemiological study is (a) To reduce or eliminate the health problem or its consequences. (b) Secondly to promote the health and well being of the population in the world.

Determinants: Determinants are factors that produce an effect, result or consequence in another factor. A determinant is a cause or factor that precipitate disease.

The determinants may be

- Physical Stresses – Excessive heat, cold and noise
- Radiation - Electromagnetic, Ultrasound, Microwave etc.
- Climate Change – Drug, acids, heavy metals, Poison and some enzymes
- Biological – Disease causing infectious agents or pathogens (Virus, Bacteria, fungi and Parasites)
- Psychological Problems: Families (Married and Divorced), households, Socioeconomic status, social networks and social support.
- Investigator can refer to any potential aetiological agent under study as a risk factor for the disease of interest, sometimes, it is named as determinant of the disease.

The main aim of epidemiology is to inform health professionals, and the public at large, in order to improve general health of public. This can be achieved by applying descriptive and aetiological analyses.

Descriptive analyses focuses on the optimal allocation of health services and targeting for the promotion of public health.

Aetiological analyses explains, what one has to do to lessen the chance of development of the disease in question.

Clinical Epidemiology

Clinical epidemiology is a branch in clinical setup, will deal more about the application of epidemiological methods in clinical trials.

It mainly focuses on evaluating, patient screening, diagnosis, treatment and prognosis, Here, different statistical tools will be applied for evaluating the accuracy of screening and diagnostic tests, identifying the level of risk associated with screening, diagnostic testing and treatment and identifying deadliness and survival probability of illness.

Population and Sampling

An epidemiological study mainly focuses on the collection of data, analysis and draw inference about the human population. In epidemiological study, investigator wish to draw the conclusions

about the population, which is termed as target population. The specific population from which the investigator collect the data is called as study population.

In some studies, the target population is defined on the basis of geographical criteria. But in majority of the epidemiological study population is based on geographical, institutional or occupational definitions. Another way of selecting the study population for epidemiological study is based on the stage or condition of the disease. Investigator goes to the diseased population, when their aim is about prevention of disease and also the study population is free from disease would be an ideal choice, when the investigator goes for follow-up studies.

If the study requires collection of any new data, we need to make groups of sample from the study population chosen for investigation. Then the investigator has to generalize from the sample to the study population and from study population to target population.

Many times the epidemiologist use the term study population as group of people from where the investigator collect the data. The rationale is that this group is the totality of those being studied, monitored ill health during a follow-up period.

CHAPTER 2

Probability and Epidemiology Study

When an experiment is performed repeatedly under similar conditions, the result we get are commonly called as outcome, may be classified as

1. It is unique or Certain
2. It is not definite, but may be one of the various possibilities depending on the experiment.

1. **It is unique or Certain:** The phenomenon under unique or certain, result that can be predicted with certainty is known as deterministic or predictable phenomenon.

   Example: If dilute sulphuric acid is added to zinc, the result we get is Hydrogen. This is certain.

2. **It is not definite, but may be one of the various possibilities depending on the experiment:** Most of the phenomenon in medical science, pharmaceutical science and in clinical studies, are deterministic in nature. However there exists number of phenomena as generated by the category 2, where the results cannot be predicted with certainty and are known as unpredictable or probabilistic phenomena. These phenomena are frequently observed in epidemiological studies.

   Example:
   (a) The sex of a baby to be born cannot be predicted with certainty.
   (b) Patient recovering completely from a particular disease after administering a treatment.

A numerical measure of uncertainty is provided by the statistical tools "Theory of probability" which is one of the most important branches of statistics.

Because of great contribution of different Mathematicians namely James Bernoulli (1650-1705) a Swiss Mathematician, De-Moivre (1667-1754), Thomas Bayers (1792 – 1761), the French Mathematician Pierre – Simon De Laplace (1749 – 1827), R.A. Fisher and the Russian mathematicians who have greatly contributed are Chebychev (1821-1894), A.Mankov (1885-1922), Khinchine and Liapounof. This subject has been developed to a great extent and this probability theory has been applied in different disciplines like Medical, Pharmaceutical and Paramedical sciences to the maximum extent. It has been applied in epidemiological studies to measure the association between factors which are considered as root cause to get disease or outcome events.

The main goal of the probability is to understand what we mean by the risk or probability of disease. Does it mean that, there is any mechanism inside our body, that decides our fate. While rejecting a particular notion the scale of randomness in epidemiological investigations, a key step in quantifying the uncertainty inherent in such studies, is also described in detail. Primarily some basic understanding of probability statement or theory is necessary.

Three fundamental components necessary to describe the probability of an occurrence are, Random experiment, Trial and Event

Random Experiment

Any experiment is said to be 'random experiment', when an experiment is conducted repeatedly under some homogeneous conditions. The result will be not unique, but may have any of the possible outcomes or one of the possible outcome may occur.

Trial: Performing a random experiment is called as trial

Example: Treating a patient with a new drug to measure the efficacy of the drug

Event: After performing an experiment, Outcome or combination of outcomes are called events

Example:

(a) When a patient is treated with a new drug, the possible outcomes may be cure or death.
(b) When two patients are treated with a new drug, the possible outcomes are Cure cure, cure death, death cure and death death.

Types of Events

Simple event: An event is said to simple event, if it corresponds to a single possible outcome of the experiment or trial.

Composite event: An event is said to be composite, if it does not correspond to a single possible outcome of the experiment or trial

Example: When two patients are treated at a time using same drug, getting either cure or death is simple event, but when both patients are cured, it can be considered as composite event

Exhaustive cases or event: The total number of possible outcomes of random experiment is called as the exhaustive event or cases for the experiment one has done.

Example:

1. When a patient is treated using a new drug, the possible outcomes of this experiment are cure or death. These two are exhaustive cases.
2. When a coin is tossed, the possible exhaustive events are head or tail.

Favorable cases or events: The number of outcomes of a random experiment, which are favorable to an investigator are termed as favorable event or events.

Example: When two patients are treated, then the favorable events are both the patients are cured.

Mutually Exclusive Events: Two or more events are said to be mutually exclusive, if the occurrence or happening of any of the event excludes or prevents the occurring or happening of any other event in the same random experiment, termed as mutually exclusive event or events.

Example: Cure of a patient prevents the occurrence of death. Here cure and death are mutually exclusive events.

Equally Likely Cases: The outcomes are said to be equally likely or equally probable, if none of them is expected to occur in preference to other.

Example: When a patient is treated, both the outcomes are equally likely, if the treatment is unbiased.

Independent Events: Two events are said to be independent, if the occurrence of one event, does not prevent the occurrence of the other event and is termed as independent events.

Example: When two patients are treated for the same type disease using same drug, then the cure of first patient does not prevent the cure of second patient.

Sample Space

The set of all possible outcomes of an experiment is termed as sample space.

Example:

1. When a coin is tossed , then the sample space S is   S = { H, T}
2. When a patient is treated, then the sample space is S= {C, D} C= Cure, D= Death.

Importance of Set Theory in Epidemiological Study

Set Theory

Set theory is used throughout mathematics. It is used as a foundation for many subfields of mathematics. In the areas pertaining to statistics, it is particularly used in probability. Much of the concepts in probability are derived from the consequences of set theory.

Definition: Set theory is the mathematical theory of well-determined collections, called sets of objects that are called members, or elements, of the set. The axioms of set theory imply the existence of a set-theoretic universe so rich that all mathematical objects can be construed as sets

Or

A set theory can be defined as a collection of well – defined objects

Example:

1. Total number of patients who are suffering from diabetics in India
2. Number of cancer patients who have been selected for clinical trial study

    In general sets are represented by the capital letters of the English alphabet, viz A, B, C….

    The commonly used symbols in set theory are

    { } – Collection of objects $\in$ – Element Belongs to a set; $\notin$ - Elements does not belongs to a set; $\cap$ - Intersection of sets ; $\cup$ - Union of sets; $\cap$- Intersection of sets

A : A is a set consisting of 5 patients suffering from asthma and 5 patients with diabetics. Then the set is written as

$$A = \{ A_1, A_2, A_3, A_4, A_5, D_1, D_2, D_3, D_4, D_5\}$$

Algebra of Sets

Union: The Union of two sets A and B is written as A∪B, the meaning of that is a set of elements which belongs to either A or B or both A and B.

Example:

A = { 1, 2, 3, 4} and B = { 3, 4,,5, 6 } then A∪B ={ 1,2,3,4,5,6}

Intersection: If A and B are two sets, then the intersection of these two sets is written A∩B.

A = { 1, 2, 3, 4} and B = { 3, 4,,5, 6 } then A∩B.={ 3,4}

Disjoint of Sets

If A and B are two sets, then they are said to be disjoint, if they do not have any common elements between them. That can be written as A∩B = Ø

Complement of a Set:

A complement of a set A is written as A^c, A^1 or $\bar{A}$

$\bar{A}$or A^c = { x : x ∉ A and x ∈ S}

Example: The set A consists of 3 patient numbers as A ={1, 3, 5} and set S consists of 6 patient numbers as S = {2,3,4,5,6,7 }

Then the A^c = {2, 4, 6}

Probability

If a random experiment results in N exhaustive, mutually exclusive and equally likely outcomes (Cases) out of which m are favorable to the happening of an event A, then the probability of occurrence of A , usually denoted by P(A) is given by

$$P(A) = \frac{\text{Number of favourable cases of A}}{\text{Exhaustive number of cases}} = \frac{m}{n}$$

OR

Probability can be defined as the ratio of the number of favorable events to the total number of possible events of a random experiment.

It can also be defined as in a random experiment, P(A) is the fraction of times the event A occurs, when the experiment is repeated many time independently and the condition is same.

Example: Suppose 20 asthma patients are treated using a drug X, the event cure (A) occurs 10 (K_A) times of the total (K) 20 experiments. Then the probability of cure (A) is written $P(A) = \frac{K_A}{K}$

= 10/20 = 0.5

Note: If the number of events which are favorable to the complementary event A, are (n – m), then by the definition of probability, the probability of non-favorable of A is defined

1. $$P\left(\overline{A}\right)=\frac{\text{Number of favourable cases of }\overline{A}}{\text{Total number of exaustive events}}$$

$$P\left(\overline{A}\right)=\frac{(N-m)}{N}=\frac{N}{N}-\frac{m}{N}=1-\frac{m}{N}=1-P(A)$$

$$P\left(\overline{A}\right)=1-P(A)$$

$$P(A)=P(\overline{A})=1$$

2. Since m and N are positive integers, $P(A) \geq 0$. The total number of favorable events always less than or equal to total number of possible events, i.e., m≤N; then $P(A) \leq 1$. Hence the P(A) lies between 0 and 1.

$$0{\leq}P(A) \leq 1.$$

3. IP(A) = 0, then it is called as impossible event or null event.

4. If P(A) = 1, then it is called as certain event.

Additional Theorem: If A, B are mutually exclusive events, then the probability of observing A or B ... is the sum of the probabilities of each event A,B

$$P(A{\cup}B) = P(A) + P(B) - P(A{\cap}B)$$

Independent Events

Two events A and B are said to be independent events, if the occurrence of one does not prevent the occurrence of other event is termed as independent event.

If A and B are two independent events, so that the probability of occurrence or non-occurrence of A is not affected by occurrence or non-occurrence of B, then we have $P(A / B) = P(A)$ and $P(B/A) = P(B)$.

Multiplicative Law

Two events A and B are independent, if and only if $P(A{\cap}B) = P(A)\,P(B)$

Note:

(a) $P(\overline{A}{\cap}B) = P(B) - P(A{\cap}B)$

(b) $P(A{\cap}\overline{B}) = P(A) - P(A{\cap}B)$

Example: The probability that a man will be alive in 30 years is 0.3 and the probability that his wife will be alive in 30 years is 0.4 What is the probability that

   (i)   Both will be alive 30 years

   (ii) Only the man will alive

   (iii) Only the woman will alive

   (iv) At least one of them will be alive.

Solution: Let

A: The man will be alive in 30 years

B: The wife will be alive in 30 years.

Given that P(A) = 0.3 and P(B) = 0.4

I

(i)   P(Both will be alive) = P(A) P(B) = (0.3)(0.4) = 0.12

(ii) P(Only man will be alive) = $P(A \cap \bar{B})$ = P(A) – P(A$\cap$B) = 0.30 – 0.12 = 0.18

OR

(iii) P(Only man will be alive) = P(A) (1 – P(B)) = 0.30 × (1 – 0.4) = 0.3 × 0.6 = 0.18

(iv) P(Only woman will be alive) = $P(\bar{A} \cap B)$ = P(B) – P(A$\cap$B) = 0.4 – 0.12 = 0.28

(v)   P(none will be alive) = $P(\bar{A} \cap \bar{B})$ = (1 – P(A)) (1 – P(B)) = (1 – 0.3) × (1 – 0.4) = 0.42

(vi) P(at least one will be alive) = 1 – P(None will be alive) = 1 – 0.42 = 0.52

Conditional Probability

If A and B two simultaneous events, where P(B/A) is the conditional probability of occurrence of event B under the condition A and P(A/B) is the conditional probability of occurrence of event A under the condition B.

Example: The data about the prevalence of Cholecystitis amongst diabetes patients and in individual with refractive errors is as listed below.

		Diabetes(D)	Refractive Error(RE)	Total
Cholecystitis	C	100	1000	1100
	$\bar{C}$	500	10000	10500
	Total	600	11000	11600

(i)   What is the probability of getting cholecystitis with the condition diabetes

(ii) What is the probability of getting cholecystitis with the condition RE

(iii) What is the probability of not getting cholecystitis ($\bar{C}$) with the condition D

(iv) What is the probability of not getting cholecystitis ($\bar{C}$) with the condition RE

Solution:

$$P(C/D) = 100/600 = 1/6$$

$$P(C/RE) = 1000/11000 = 1/11$$

$$P(\bar{C}/D) = 500/600 = 5/6$$

$$P(\bar{C}/RE) = 10000/11000 = 10/11$$

Note:

1. If A and B are the two possible outcomes of an experiment then

   (a) $P(A \cap B) = P(A) + P(B) - P(A \cup B)$

   (b) $P(A \cup B) = P(A) + P(B) - P(A \cap B)$

Example 2: A investigator makes research on a sample of size 125 with Age <65 and Age>65 are classified according age, CHD problem and Diabetic problem as listed below.

	Age ≤ 65		Age > 65	
	Diabetic	NO Diabetic	Diabetic	NO Diabetic
CHD	27	20	18	10
No. CHD	18	10	12	10

   (i)   What is the probability of having CHD ?

   (ii) If age is > 65 and is a diabetic, what is the probability that patient will have CHD?

   (iii) What is the conditional probability patient having CHD and also patent is having diabetic?

   (iv) Are the events CHD and Diabetic are independent?. Comment

Solution:

Let A – be the patients with CHD, B – Patient with diabetic,

   C – Patients with age > 65

For the given data $P(A) = \dfrac{27 + 20 + 18 + 10}{125} = 0.6; , P(B) = \dfrac{27 + 18 + 18 + 12}{125} = 0.6, P(C) = 0.4$

$$P(A \cap B) = P[\text{Having CHD and Diabetic}] = \frac{27 + 18}{125} = \frac{45}{125}$$

$$P(B \cap C) = P[\text{Having diabetic and age} > 65] = \frac{18 + 12}{125} = \frac{30}{125}$$

$$P(A \cap B \cap C) = P[\text{Having CHD , Diabetic and Age} > 65] = \frac{18}{125}$$

   (i) $P(\text{Having CHD}) = P(A) = 0.6$

   (ii) $P(\text{CHD/, Diabetic, Age>65}) =$

$$P(A \backslash B \cap C) = \frac{P(A \cap B \cap C)}{P(B \cap C)} = (18/125)/(30/125) = 0.6$$

   (iii) P(What is the conditional probability patient having CHD and also patent is having diabetic?)

$$- P(A/B) = \frac{P(A \cap B)}{P(B)} = (45/125)/(75/125). - 0.6$$

(iv) P(The events CHD and Diabetic are independent?)

$\quad$ = P(A∩B) = 9/125 and P(A) × P(B) = 3/5 × 3/5 = 9/25

Since P(A∩B) = P(A) × P(B), then A and B statistically independent.

Data given below is about infant mortality or deaths and live for one year when mother is smoker and non smoker. Find the conditional probability of death due to smoking and non-smoking.

		Mother Status		
Infant Mortality	**Smokers**	**NON Smokers**	**Total**
Death	200	300	500
Live at 1 Year	1000	2000	3000
Total	1200	2300	3500

Solution:

A - Death

B – Smoker

P(A&B)	200/3500	0.0571
P(B)	1200/3500	0.3429
P(A/B) = P(A&B)/P(B)	0.0571/0.3429	0.1667

A - Death

C = Non Smoker

P(A&C)	300/3500	0.0857
P(C)	2300/3500	0.6571
P(A/C)	0.0857/0.6571	0.1304

Conditional Probabilities

We have discussed the probability that a randomly selected infant dies within 1year of birth for the population summarized in. But what if we want to know this probability for important subgroups of the population?

For example, Role of Probability in Observational Studies interested in the probability of death within a year after birth due to the association of an unmarried mother or for a normal birth weight infant. In both the case the investigator is looking for the conditional probability of the outcome.

If A is considered as infants' death within a year from the date of birth, and B represent the randomly chosen event of birth due to the unmarried mother, then the P(A\B) is the probability children dies within a year due to unmarried mother.

To compute the conditional probability $P(A|B)$, we have to calculate the long run fraction of times the event A occurs among events where B also occurs.

Consider a series K independent equivalent experiments, let $K_{A\&B}$ denotes the total number experiments where both events A and B occur. Then the fraction of times that event A occurs amongst those experiments where event B occurs is written as $K_{(A\&B)}/K_B$.

Thus, the conditional probability $P(A|B)$ is the "long run" value of $K_{(A\&B)}/K_B$. But, by dividing both the numerator and denominator of this expression by K, we see that this conditional probability is given by the "long run" value of $K_{A\&B}/K$ divided by the "long run" value of K_B/K. More simply,

$$P(A/B) = \frac{P(A \,\&\, B)}{P(B)}$$

An immediate consequence of this expression is a formulation for the probability of the composite event, A and B:

$$P(A\&B) = P(A|B) \times P(B))$$

By reversing the roles of the events A and B, it follows that $P(B|A)=P(A\&B)/P(A)$ so that

$$P(A\&B) = P(B|A) \times P(A))$$

When we select a random member of a population, the probability that the selected individual has a specific characteristic is just the population proportion of individuals with this attribute.

That is, for a randomly selected individual, the conditional probability that an individual has characteristic A, given that they possess characteristic B, namely, $P(A|B)$, is the population proportion of individuals with characteristic A amongst the subpopulation who have characteristic B.

Thus, A denotes death in the first year and B denotes having an unmarried mother, then $P(A|B)$, the conditional probability of death within a year of birth, given that the infant has an unmarried mother, is

	Infant mortality between mother's marital status and birth weight		
	Marital status of Mother		
Infant Mortality	**Married**	**Not Married**	**Total**
Death	15200	17500	3270
Live for one year	1180150	2978321	4158471
Total	1195350	2995821	4191171

$P(A) = 15200/(1180150+15200) = 0.01272$ or 12 death per 1000

$P(A\&B) = 15200/4191171 = 0.003627$, $P(B) = 1195350/4191171 = 0.2852$

$P(A\backslash B) = P(A\&B)/P(B) = 0.003627/0.2852 = 0.0127$

It is important to note that the conditional probability of $A|B$ is quite different from that of $B|A$.

Inference made on the Basis of Estimated Probability

When an investigator randomly selects sample from the population of size n possessing the characteristic A. Then we can write the probability of A as $P = P(A)$

$$P = P = \frac{nA}{n} \frac{\text{Number of favourable of favourable of A}}{\text{Total number of possible event}}$$, generally P will be written as $\hat{P}$, then the

variance can be obtained by the equation $\frac{\hat{P}(1-\hat{P})}{n}$, then the confidence interval can be constructed

using the equation

$$P\left(\frac{\left|\hat{P} - P\right|}{\sqrt{\frac{\hat{P}(1-\hat{P})}{n}}} \leq Z\alpha/2 \right)$$

Then by implying this equation we get the confidence interval as

$$\hat{P} - Z\alpha/2\sqrt{\frac{\hat{P}(1-\hat{P})}{n}} \leq P \leq \hat{P} + Z\alpha/2$$

Example: Consider a sample of size 100 infants were drawn from the population, where 35 infants births are associated with unmarried women. Construct 95 confidence interval for the birth of 35 infants who are associated unmarried women.

Solution: $\hat{P} = 35/100 = 0.35$

Then the confidence interval for 95% confidence is

$$\hat{P} \pm Z\alpha/2\sqrt{\frac{\hat{P}(1-\hat{P})}{n}}$$

$$= 0.35 \pm 1.96\sqrt{\frac{0.35(1-0.65)}{100}}$$

$$= (0.272, 0.428)$$

Joint and Marginal Probability

Consider two discrete random variables X and Y.

Let us consider that X assume the m variables $x_1, x_2, \ldots\ldots x_m$ and Y assumes the n-variables say $y_1, y_2, \ldots y_n$.

Let the probability of order pairs of these two discrete random variables X and Y be (x_i, y_j)

$$i = 1, 2, 3 - - - - - m$$

$j = 1,2,3- - - - - - -n$, then probability $P_{ij} = P(x = x_i$ and $Y = y_j) = P(x_i, y_j)$

The function $P(x, y)$ which is defined for any ordered pair (x, y) is called as joint probability and that can also be represented in table as

X〔Y〕	x_1	x_2		x_m	Total
y_1	P_{11}	P_{21}		P_{m1}	P_1^I
y_2	P_{12}	P_{22}		P_{m2}	P_2^I
y_n	P_{1n}	P_{2n}		P_{mn}	P_m^I
Total	$P1$	$P2$		Pm	1

By using the joint probability of discrete random variables X and Y, then the marginal probability function X can be written as

$$P_i = P(X=x_i) = P_{i1} + P_{i2}+ - - - - - - - +Pim)\ (i=1,2\ ,3\ ----m)$$

$$= \sum_{j=1}^{n} P_{ij}$$

The set of values $\{xi, yj\}$,$i= 1,2,3,-----m$ gives the marginal probability distribution of X

Similarly $P_j^1 = P(Y = y_j) = P1j +P2j +- - - - - Pmj\ (j = 1,2,3\ ----n)$

$$= \sum_{j=1}^{n} P_{ij}$$

This gives the marginal probability function of Y and the set values $\{Y, P_j^1\}$; $j = 1,2,3----$ ngives the marginal probability distribution of Y. That can be written as $\sum_i \sum_j P_{ij}$

Note: Two random variables which are named as X and Y are said to be independent, if and only if their joint probability function is equal to the product of their marginal probability functions.

$$P(X = x_i \cap y_i = Y) = PX=x_i), P(Y = y_i),\ ie\ P_{ij}= P_iXp_j$$

Example: Obtain the Joint probability between disease status and exposure and also obtain Marginal Probability of disease status due to exposure,

Solution:

		Disease Status		
		Cancer	No Cancer	Total
Exposure of Smoking	Smoker	12	200	212
	Non Smoker	8	100	108
	Total	20	300	320

Joint Probability

Joint Probability of P(Smokers and Cancer)	12/320	0.0375	
Joint Probability of P(Non Smokers and Cancer)	08/320	0.025	
Joint Probability of P(Smokers and No Cancer)	200/320	0.625	
Joint Probability of P(Non smokers and No Cancer)	100/320	0.3125	
		1.0000	

Marginal Probability

The Marginal Probability P(Cancer)	20/320	0.0625
The Marginal Probability P(No Cancer)	300/320	0.9375
		1

Conditional Probability

Conditional Probability P(Cancer/Smoking)	12/212	0.06
Conditional Probability P(No Cancer/Smoking)	200/212	0.94
Total		1.00
Conditional Probability P(Cancer/ No Smoking)	08/108	0.07
Conditional Probability P(No. Cancer/ No Smoking)	100/108	0.93
Total		1.00

Example:

Two industries which are manufacturing some medical devices, which are used to carry out operation of heart patients. Each medical device is classified as 0, 1, 2, 3 according to their manufacturing defects. The joint probability for this is as listed in the table.

Manufacturing Industries	Number of Defects			
	0	1	2	3
X	0.1250	0.0625	0.1875	0.1250
Y	0.0625	0.0625	0.1250	0.2500

(a) What is the probability that no defect in the medical device manufacture by the Company X.

(b) What is the probability that 2 or More defects of medical devices, which are manufactured by X.

(c) What is the Probability one or more defect of medical devices, which are manufactured by Y.

Solution:

	0	1	2	3	Total
X	0.125	0.0625	0.1875	0.125	0.5
Y	0.0625	0.0625	0.125	0.25	0.5
Total	0.1875	0.125	0.3125	0.375	1

(a) $P[\text{X/No defect}] = \dfrac{P(X \cap D = 0)}{P(D = 0)} = 0.125/0.1875 = 0.6667$

(b) $P[X/D \geq 2] = \dfrac{P(X \cap D \geq 2)}{P(D \geq 2)} = (0.1875 + 0.1250)/(0.3125 + 0.375) = 0.3125/0.6875$

$= 0.4545$

(c) $P[Y/D \geq 2] = \dfrac{P(X \cap D \geq 1)}{P(D \geq 1)} = (0.0625 + 0.1250 + 0.2500) / (0.1250 + 0.3125 + 0.3750)$

$= 0.5385$

Baye's Theorem

This theorem was derived by British Mathematician Thomas Baye's (1702 – 1761), to measure probability and draw statistical inference. This theorem is more useful for inverse probability.

Statement: If an event A can only occur in conjunction with one of the n-mutually exclusive and exhaustive events E_1, E_2, ---------E_n, and if A actually happens, then the probability that it was preceded by a particular event E_i (I = 1,2, - -- n) is given by

$$P(E_i / A) = \frac{P(A \cap E_i)}{\Sigma P(E_i).P(A / E_i)}$$

Example: A canteen in a hospital provides two types of special dishes A and B to its patients consisting of 60% men and 40% women. 80% 0f men patients order for dish A and the remaining men patients order for B. 70% of women patients order for B and the rest of them order for dish A. Obtain the ratio of A to B should the canteen prepare the two dishes.

Solution:

Let A : Patient order for food A

Let B : Patient order for B

M : The male patient

W: The Female Patient

Given that

$$P(M) = 0.6 \qquad P(W) = 0.4$$
$$P(A/M) = 0.8 \qquad P(B/M) = 0.2$$
$$P(A/W) = 0.3 \qquad P(B/W) = 0.7$$

The food ordered by men or women can be written as

$$A = (A \cap M) \cap M) (A \cup W)$$
$$P(A) = P((A \cap M) \cup (A \cup W))$$
$$= P(A \cap M) + P(A \cap W)$$
$$= P(M)P(A/M) + P(W) P(A/W)$$
$$= 0.6 \times 0.8 + 0.4 \times 0.3 = 0.48 + 0.12 = 0.60$$
$$P(B) = P((B \cap M) \cup (B \cup W))$$
$$= P(B \cap M) + (B \cap W))$$
$$= P(M)P(B/M) + P(W) P(B/W)$$
$$= 0.6 \times 0.2 + 0.4 \times 0.7 = 0.12 + 0.28 = 0.40$$

A screening test can be considered as a preventative measure – to detect the health problem or disease in someone that doesn't yet have signs or symptoms. The screening test helps for early detection of disease and helps in reducing the risk of disease, or detect the condition of patients in the beginning and helps to treat the disease most effectively.

Application to Screening Study

Imagine a study evaluating a new test that screens people for a disease. Every individual taking the test either has or does not have the disease. The test outcome when it is positive, then that individual subject can be included in the diseased group and if the result is negative then that individual will be included in not having disease group. The test results for each subject may or may not match the subject's actual status. In that case we different groups as listed below.

True positive: Sick people correctly identified as sick,

False positive: Healthy people incorrectly identified as sick

True negative: Healthy people correctly identified as healthy

False negative: Sick people incorrectly identified as healthy

In general, Positive = identified and negative = rejected. Therefore:

True positive = correctly identified

False positive = incorrectly identified

True negative = correctly rejected

False negative = incorrectly rejected

Sensitivity and Specificity

Sensitivity and **specificity** are statistical method to measure the performance of two test which are classified binary and in biostatistics it is called as classification function and most widely used in medical profession.

Sensitivity that measures the proportion of actual positives that are correctly identified after performing the diagnostic test (e.g., the percentage of sick people who have been identified as having the disease or showing the positive report).

Specificity measures the proportion of actual negatives that are correctly identified after performing the diagnostic test (e.g., the percentage of healthy people who have been identified as not having the condition or showing the negative report).

Test Result↓	Status of Disease		Total
	Disorder	**No Disorder**	**Total**
Positive test Result	True Positive (TP)	False Positive (FP)	TP + FP
Negative test Result	False Negative (FN)	True Negative (TN)	FN + TN
Total	TP + FN	FP + TN	

Sensitivity = TP/TP + FN

Specificity = TN/FP + TN

PPV = TP/TP + FP

NPV = TN/FN + TN

Using those four we calculate sensitivity, specificity, and positive and negative predictive

CHAPTER 3

Mathematical Measures and Epidemiological Studies

Mathematical Measurements in Epidemiological Studies

Epidemiological study mainly focuses, on some of the important mathematical measurements like1.Rate 2. Ratio3. Proportion 4. Morbidity and 5. Mortality.

Rate: This is one of the mathematical tool, that will be used to measure the occurrence of some particular types of events, like getting or developing a particular disease or number of deaths occurred in a population during a given period of time. It can be considered as risk of developing particular condition.

The rate comprises the following elements like numerator, denominator, time specification and multiplier. The time specification refers to a calendar year.

In general the rate will be expressed per 100 or 10000, 100000, according to our convenience to avoid that fractional value.

$$\text{Birth Rate} = \frac{\text{Number of births in one year}}{\text{Total population of the middle year}}$$

Ratio

The important mathematical measurement, which will be used to measure the disease frequency is ratio. This explains the relation in terms of size between two random numbers or quantities. Broadly ratio is the result of dividing one quantity by another, it can be written in the form as x:y or $\text{Ratio} = \dfrac{x}{y}$.

Example **1:** The ratio of white blood cells relative to the red cells is written as 1:600 or $\text{Ratio} = \dfrac{1}{600}$.

Example **2:** If a and b are similar quantities, measured from different groups or under different circumstances, then ratio can be written as

$$\text{Ratio} = \frac{a}{b} = \frac{\text{Male smokers}}{\text{Female smokers}}$$

The ratio will be positive and may be greater than 1.

Proportion: A proportion is a ratio which indicates the relation in magnitude of a part of the whole. The numerator is always included in the denominator. Generally proportion will be expressed as a percentage.

$$\text{Proportion} = \frac{\text{Number of children with asthma problem at a certain time}}{\text{Total number of children in a particular village at the same time}}$$

OR

Proportion is a number used to describe a group of people according to a dichotomous or binary characteristic under investigation.

Measurement of Mortality

Mortality is defined as death due to some exposure. Traditionally and universally most epidemiological studies begins with mortality. Mortality data are relatively easy to obtain and in many countries, reasonably accurate. Mortality, rather than morbidity is the outcome which will be recorded. Many countries have routine systems for collecting mortality data. Event notification arises from routine statistics, rather than making any special observation, Mortality data provide the starting point for many epidemiological studies. In fact they are the major resources for epidemiologist to carry out their research work.

Mortality Rates and Ratios

The mortality conditions of a population are studied by measuring the following mortality rates.
1. Crude death rate
2. Specific death rate
3. Standardized death rate

Crude Death Rate

The simplest measure of mortality is crude death rate. Crude death is the ratio of the total death due to so many diseases of some specified year to the total population, multiplied by 1000, it is written as

$$\text{Crude Death Rate} = \frac{\text{Total number of deaths in a given locality during the year}}{\text{Annual mean population}} \times 1000$$

$\text{CDR} = \dfrac{\Sigma D}{\Sigma P} \times 1000$, ΣD = Total deaths in a year and, ΣP = Total mean population. This crude death rate gives the level of mortality of the entire population. It is easily and quickly computed. But there are certain limitations of crude death rate, because these data's are not much appropriate for making comparison between two populations. The crude rate between two populations may be same, but we may find some wide differences in the age and racial composition, occupational pattern, density, sanitary conditions etc, between these two populations.

The crude death rate may be higher in one population, because of relatively high aged people in that community, through the mortality at various ages may be low.

Specific Death Rate

A death rate can be calculated on the basis of a specified segment of the population and is called as specific death rate.

Death rates may be specific with respect to age, sex, deaths due to special cause (Cancer, ulcer, small pox) or due to some other characteristics.

Specific death Rate =

$$\frac{\text{Specific deaths in a specific section of the population of a given area during a given year}}{\text{Mid year population of the specific section}}$$

Specific death rates can help everyone to identify particular group at risk for preventive action. It is more useful for the comparisons between different causes within the same population. Thus these rates can be compared from one population to the other or from one time period to another within a population. Nevertheless, the specific deaths rates are most meaningful as measure of mortality prevailing in a community.

Standardized Death Rates

As the specific death rate compute for different segments of the population, these rates are not very useful when, we wish to make comparison between mortality prevailing in two countries. It is more meaningful for examining the specific death rates, than the crude rate, This specific rates are more meaningful to examine specific rate like – cause or disease specific (like tuberculosis, cancer, accident) and also useful for related like specific age, sex etc. This can also be made specific for other factors or variables like income, religion , race, housing etc. This specific rate gives us an accurate pictures of mortality between males and females at each age. This also helps us to compare between different causes within the population.

But these rates not very useful when we wish to make comparison between mortality prevailing in two countries. For a meaning compression to do medical survey, or research, we need a single index for comparison purpose. The specific death rate fails to reveal the real mortality. In this case the crude death rate is to be adjusted to allow for the known differences in the age comparison of the populations involved. A number of methods which are designed for the adjustment, which are called as adjusted rates, standardized rates or corrected rates. The specific death rates are combined by a process, known as standardization to make adjustments for age composition of population. Standardization is done in order to eliminate the effect of age composition, so that any comparison will show the real difference in mortality in two populations.

The standardization is carried out by two methods, They are named as (a) Direct method, (b) Standardization

Direct Method: According to this method, the population which is taken form a locality or region is taken as standard population. The specific death rates of different age groups of the population are multiplied by the respective age-group of standard population. The respective result of each age-group is totaled up and the total is divided by the total of the standard population. It is written as

$$SDR = \frac{\Sigma Px / D_i}{Ps}$$

Here Px = standard population for different age groups.

D$_i$ = Specific death rate of local population.

This method is feasible only, when the actual specific rates in subgroups of the observed population are available, along with the numbers of individuals in each subgroup.

Indirect Method: In case of the specific death rates, are not known, for the population in question and the age composition is given, then we apply indirect method for standardization. In this method, the standard is set for specific rates, rather than for age composition of the population. For the computation of SDR for the local population, the specific death rates, which are taken as standard are multiplied with the corresponding age groups of the local population. The sum of the product is obtained, in turn that total is divided by total local population, which will give index death rate for local population. The index death rate of the population $= \dfrac{\Sigma \dfrac{P}{lx} DS}{\Sigma Pl}$

Pl = Local population for various age groups

Ds = Specific age death rates of standard population

The crude death rate of the standard population is computed by using the equation

$$\text{CDR of standard population} = \frac{\Sigma P_s \times Ds}{\Sigma P_s}$$

Ps = Standard population for different age groups.

Then correction factor is obtained by dividing CDR of standard population by the index death of local population.

$$\text{Correction factor} = \frac{\text{CDR of standard population}}{\text{Index death rate of local population}}$$

$$= \frac{\dfrac{\Sigma P_s \times D_s}{\Sigma P_s}}{\dfrac{\Sigma \dfrac{Pl}{lx} Ds}{\Sigma Pl}}$$

Then the standardized death rate of the local population is obtained by multiplying the crude death rate of the local population is multiplied by the correction factor.

$$\text{SDR (Local population)} = \text{CDR (Local Population)} \times \text{C.F}$$

Measurement of Morbidity

Morbid: Illness, sickness or morbid condition is defined as the deviation from a state of Physical or mental well-being as a result of disease, injury or impairment.

OR

Morbidity can also be defined as "Any departure of subjective or objective, from a state of physiological well-being. The term used equivalent to the terms of sickness, illness, disability etc.

The average duration per case or the disability rate, which is the average number of days of disability per person, may serve as a measure of the duration of illness.

Incidence and Prevalence

The disease incidence and Prevalence both represent proportion of a population determined to the disease at certain times. Before we give an informal definition, we should note the time scale used must be defined carefully. The time scales used could be defined as

1. The age of individual
2. Duration of exposure to a specific factor
3. Calendar time or
4. Time from diagnosis

Incidence

The incidence is defined as "the number of new cases occurring in a defined population during a specified period of time.

OR

Incidence tells how often an event occurs in a population over a period of time, such as a week, a month, a year etc.

Incidence Rate =

$$\frac{\text{Number of persons who developed the disease over a period defined period of time}}{\text{Number of persons intially without the disease, who were followed for the defined period of time}} \times K$$

The value of K depends on the magnitude of the numerator. The base of 1000 is used when it is convenient, but 100 can be used, when the disease is more common and 10000 can be the diseases which are very rare. This rate, which measures the degree to which all the new cases are occurring in the community, is more useful in helping to take initiation to take preventive measures. This measure of incidence rate is most useful for chronic and acute diseases.

Example: If there had been 500 new cases with a particular disease, like cancer in a population of size 30,000, in a year (defined period) due to the risk factor smoke, then the incidence rate is

$$\text{Incidence Rate} = \frac{500}{30000} \times 1000 = 16.7 \text{ per 1000 per year.}$$

Uses of Incidence Rate

Incidence rate can be considered as a health status indicator and is more useful for taking action like (a) To control the disease (b) To carry our research into aeitiology and Pathogenesis, distribution of diseases, and efficacy of preventive and therapeutics measures.

Prevalence

The term prevalence of a disease is the proportion of a defined population at risk, for disease that is affected by it at a specified point on the time scale.

The term "PREVALENCE" refers specially to all current cases (old or New) existing at a given point in time or over a period of time in a given population. A broader definition of prevalence is defined as the ratio of diseased persons at the time of investigation, to the total number of persons examined at that period.

$$\text{Prevalence} = \frac{\text{Total number of cases, new or old, existing at a point in time}}{\text{Total population at that point in time}} \times K$$

Where K is selected with the same criteria, which are considered in calculation of incidence rate.

It also can be defined as the total number of all individuals, who have an attribute or disease at a particular time (or during a particular period) divided by the population at risk having the attribute or disease at this point in time or midway through the period.

Advantages: The simplest use of this measure of disease occurring is their comparison across subgroups that have experienced different levels of exposure.

Example: One can compare the prevalence rate of cancer between adult male who are smokers against adult males who have never smoked.

Disadvantages: To investigate the etiology of a disease, not only depend on initiation, but also on the duration of disease.

Relationship between Prevalence and Incidence: The prevalence depends on 2-factors, the incidence and duration of illness. Under the assumption that the population is stable, and incidence and durations are not changeable, then the relationship between I and P can be written using the mathematical equation $P = I \times D$, where I = Incidence and D = Average (Mean) duration.

If we know the prevalence, then it is possible for us to compute incidence using the equation

$$I = P/D$$

Similarly duration can also be obtained when P and I are known $D = P/I$.

The Equation $P = I \times D$ indicates that the longer the duration of the disease, the greater its prevalence.

Mathematical equation to measure association between Disease – Exposure

For many disease, the health profession still not able to identify the disease factor for many diseases.

Example: Coronary Heart disease, Cancer, Peptic ulcer, Mental disorder etc. In general the word aetiology is discussed in terms of Risk Factors.

The risk factor can be defined as

  (a) Attribute or exposure that is significantly associated with the development of a disease.
  (b) A determinant that can be modified by intervention, thereby reducing the possibility of occurrence of disease or any other particular outcomes.

Estimation of Risk

Relative Risk

The estimation of disease risk associated with exposure is obtained by an index known as relative risk.

The relative risk is defined as the ratio between incidence of disease among exposed persons and incidence among non-exposed. It can computed using the equation

$$\text{Relative risk} = \frac{\text{Incidence in expose group}}{\text{Incidence in non - exposed group}}$$

Factor	Diseased		Total
	Yes	No	
Exposed	a	b	a + b
Non-exposed	c	d	c + d
Total	a + c	b + d	N = a + b + c + d

$$\text{Relative Risk} = \text{RR} = \frac{\dfrac{a}{a+b}}{\dfrac{c}{c+d}}$$

The relative risk can also be defined by using the incidence proportions. If D is outcome associated with a binary risk factor E (Exposure) and $\overline{E}$ (Not exposed), then relative risk RR can be defined as $\text{RR} = \dfrac{P(D / E)}{P(D / \overline{E})}$. The relative risk always must be nonnegative number, when the RR = 1, this implies that $P(D/E) = P(D/\overline{E})$ or D and E are independent. Other way we can say that no effects of risk factor. When the RR > 1, then there is a greater risk or risk is more harmful. Is RR = 3, then we can say that people exposed have a risk of getting a particular disease, that is approximately three times the risk of those subjects who are unexposed to the risk factor. When the RR < 1 indicate there is beneficial effect of the exposed factor.

Example: In a sample of size 117 subject or persons, 88 were exposed to the risk factor (Smoking) and 29 were not exposed to the risk factor (Smoking), the data listed in the table provides the information about the number of people who have suffering from cancer (Case) and not suffering from cancer (Control). Compute the relative risk and verify the effect of Relative Risk.

Factor	Diseased Status		Total
	Case (Cancer is Present)	Control (No Cancer)	
Smoking	33(a)	55 (b)	a + b = 88
Non-Smoking	2(c)	27d	c + d = 29
Total	a + c = 35	b + d	N = a + b + c + d = 117

Solution:

$$\text{Relative Risk} = RR = \frac{\dfrac{a}{a+b}}{\dfrac{c}{c+d}} = \frac{\dfrac{33}{88}}{\dfrac{2}{29}} = \frac{0.375}{0.068} = 5.514$$

$$RR > 1 = 5.514$$

This indicates that there is good association between lung cancer and smoking and it indicating the negative effect of smoking or smoking is more dangerous.

Odds Ratio

With the help of case-control study, the investigator can derive the odds ratio, which measures the strength of association between the risk factor and outcomes. The computation of odds ratio mainly depends on three important assumptions:

(a) The disease which is selected for study or clinical research must be relatively very rare.
(b) The cases selected for study or clinical research must be representative of those with disease and
(c) The controls must be representative of the subgroup without disease.

$$OR = \frac{\dfrac{a}{a+b}}{\dfrac{c}{c+d}}$$

In general $a + b \simeq b$ and $c + d \simeq d$

$$\text{Then the OR} = \frac{\dfrac{a}{b}}{\dfrac{c}{d}} = \frac{ad}{bc}$$

Just like the relative risk the ODD's ratio measures the association by comparing the odds of D (disease) between the exposed (E) and unexposed groups ($\overline{E}$) which are chosen from the defined population. Then the OR can be defined as

$$OR = \frac{\dfrac{P\left(\dfrac{D}{E}\right)}{P\left(\dfrac{D}{\bar{E}}\right)}}{\dfrac{P\left(\dfrac{D}{\bar{\bar{E}}}\right)}{P\left(\dfrac{D}{\bar{\bar{E}}}\right)}} = \frac{\dfrac{P\left(\dfrac{D}{E}\right)}{P\left(\dfrac{\text{Not D}}{E}\right)}}{\dfrac{P\left(\dfrac{D}{\text{Not E}}\right)}{P\left(\dfrac{\text{Not D}}{\text{Not E}}\right)}}$$

When the computed value of OR = 1 indicates that D and E are independent, if OR > 1, this indicates there is greater risk of D with the exposure or due to the exposure E, than an unexposed ($\bar{E}$), then the reverse is also true when OR < 1, that indicates that there is a lower risk D due to the exposure E.

In a sample of size 117 subject or persons, 88 were exposed to the risk factor (Smoking) and 29 were not exposed to the risk factor (Smoking), the data listed in the table provides the information about the number of people who have been suffering from cancer (Case) and not suffering from cancer (Control). Compute the ODD Ratio and verify the effect of ODD Ratio.

Factor	Diseased Status		Total
	Case (Cancer is Present)	Control (No Cancer)	
Smoking	33(a)	55 (b)	a + b = 88
Non-Smoking	2(c)	27d	c + d = 29
Total	a + c = 35	b + d	N = a + b + c + d = 117

OR = ad/bc = (33×27)/(2×55) = 8.1

Computation of ODDs Ratio Using SPSS

Risk Estimate				
Values		Value	95% Confidence Interval	
			Lower	Upper
2.00	Odds Ratio for ROW (2 / .)	.[a]		
27.00	Odds Ratio for ROW (2 / .)	.[a]		
33.00	Odds Ratio for ROW (1 / .)	.[a]		
55.00	Odds Ratio for ROW (1 / .)	.[a]		
Total	Odds Ratio for ROW (1 / 2)	8.100	1.808	36.293
	For cohort COL = 1	5.438	1.390	21.275
	For cohort COL = 2	.671	.555	.812
	N of Valid Cases	117		
a. No statistics are computed because ROW and COL are constants.				

$$\text{OR} = \frac{\left(\dfrac{P\dfrac{D}{E}}{P\left(\dfrac{\overline{D}}{E}\right)}\right)}{\left(\dfrac{P\left(\dfrac{D}{\overline{E}}\right)}{P\left(\dfrac{\overline{D}}{\overline{E}}\right)}\right)} = \frac{\left(\dfrac{33/88}{55/88}\right)}{\left(\dfrac{2/29}{27/29}\right)} = \frac{\left(\dfrac{0.375}{0.625}\right)}{\left(\dfrac{0.0689}{0.9310}\right)} = 8.10$$

Note:

Measures of Association for Two-Level Nominal Exposure and Outcome Variables

When an investigator collects data after performing different types studies will be tabulated in 2×2 with exposure and outcome variables, then the Odd Ratio, Relative Risk and Rate Ratio for different types studies can obtained using different equations as explained below.

Exposed	Disease		Total
	Yes	No	
YES	a	b	a + b
NO	c	d	c + d
Total	a + c	b + d	N = a + b + c + d

Concordance and Discordance

Consider a $2 \times k$ table as listed below

	Column Level					
Row	1	2	3	....	k	Total
1	a_1	a_2	a_3	....	a_k	A
2	b_1	b_2	b_3	....	b_k	B
Total	n_1	n_2	n_3	....	n_k	N

The number of concordance can be obtained using the equation

$$C = a_1(b_2 + b_3 + \text{----}b_k) + a_2(b_3 + b_4 + \text{------}b_k) + \text{------------} + a_{k-1}b_k$$

The Discordance can be obtained by the equation

$$D = b_1(a_2 + a_3 + \text{----} + a_k) + b_2(a_3 + a_4 + \text{------} + a_k) + \text{------------} + b_{k-1}a_k$$

Then the generalized Odd ratio can be obtained by the equation

$$\theta = \frac{C}{D}$$

In case of 2×2 –contingency table with Case and Control as listed below

Disease Status

Risk Factor	Case	Control
Exposed	a	b
Not Exposed	c	d

The number of case-control pairs with different exposure histories (ad + bc); among ad pairs with an exposed case and bc pairs with an exposed control. The ratio ad/bc is the odds of finding a pair with an exposed case among discordant pairs (a discordant pair is a case – control pair with different exposure histories).

Analysis_Chi-square_Mantel Haenszel and Meta-analysis – Odds Ratio

The Mantel-Haenszel analysis provides two closely related pieces of information. First, it provides statistical tests of whether the odds ratios are equal (homogeneous) or unequal (heterogeneous) across strata. Second, it provides an estimate of the odds ratio of the exposure variable, adjusted for the strata variable.

Case-control studies of dichotomous outcomes (e.g., Cured or not-cured) can be represented by arranging the observed counts into fourfold (2 × 2) tables. The separation of data into different tables or strata represents a sub-grouping, like different age groups. This type of stratification sometimes used to reduce confounding. A confounder or confounding variable, is a variable that may be associated with disease or exposure of both.

The Mantel-Haenszel method provides a pooled odds ratio across the strata of fourfold tables. Meta-analysis is used to investigate the combination or interaction of a group of independent studies, for example a series of fourfold tables from similar studies conducted at different centers.

For a single stratum odds ratio is estimated as follows:

		Exposure	
		Exposed	Not -Exposed
Outcome	Cases	a	b
	Controls	c	d

The odds Ratio of is obtained by the equation OR = (ad)/(bc)

When different strata's are considered, then using the Mantel-Haenszel method the pooled Odd Ratio is obtained at different level of confounder using the equation

$$ORMH = \frac{\sum_{i=1}^{k}\left(\dfrac{a_i d_i}{n_i}\right)}{\sum_{i=1}^{k}\left(\dfrac{b_i c_i}{n_i}\right)} \quad \text{where } n_i = a_i + b_i + c_i + d_i$$

Example: A study was conducted to investigate the relationship between the heart attack

***Example* 1:** The data given below is about the number of deaths/survivors in the study population according to pneumonia infection and the different age group as confounder. Compute pooled Odd Ratio by applying Mantel-Haenszel method.

		Age<60 (n = 116)	
		Exposed	**Not -Exposed**
Pneumonia Infection	Positive	10	30
	Negative	20	70

and

		Age≥ 60 (n = 111)	
		Exposed	**Not -Exposed**
Pneumonia Infection	Positive	31	26
	Negative	23	31

Solution:

		Age<60 (n = 130)		
		Exposed	**Not -Exposed**	**Total**
Pneumonia Infection	Positive	10	30	40
	Negative	20	70	90
	Total	30	100	130

$a_1 d_1 / n_1 = (10 \times 70)/130 = 5.38$

$b_1 c_1 / n_1 = (30 \times 20)/130 = 4.62$

		Age < 60 (n = 116)		
		Exposed	**Not -Exposed**	**Total**
Pneumonia Infection	Positive	31	56	87
	Negative	25	35	60
	Total	56	91	147

$a_2 d_2 / n_2 = (31 \times 35)/147 = 7.38$

$c_2 d_2 / n_2 = (56825)/147 = 9.52$

$$OR_{MH} = \frac{\sum_{i=1}^{k} \left(\dfrac{a_i d_i}{n_i} \right)}{\sum_{i=1}^{k} \left(\dfrac{b_i c_i}{n_i} \right)} \text{ where } n_i = a_i + b_i + c_i + d_i$$

$$= \frac{\dfrac{a_1 d_1}{n_1} + \dfrac{a_2 d_2}{n_2}}{\dfrac{b_1 c_1}{n_1} + \dfrac{b_2 c_2}{n_2}} = \frac{5.38 + 7.38}{4.62 + 9.52} = 5.91$$

***Example* 2:** Patients are stratified according to their age and they are classified by their disease status. The data listed in the table gives information about the association between the hypertension (risk Factor) and obstructive coronary artery disease (OCAD). Compute Odd ratio by applying the Mantel-Haenszel method

Stratified Group-I (Age ≤ 55)

Risk Factor(Hypertension)	Cases(OCAD)	Control (OCAD)	Total
Present	25	12	37
Absent	20	10	30
Total	45	22	67

Stratified Group-I (Age > 55)

Risk Factor(Hypertension)	Cases(OCAD)	Control (OCAD)	Total
Present	55	18	37
Absent	22	10	30
Total	77	28	105

$a_1 d_1/n_1 = 25 \times 10/76 = 3.73, \quad d_2 d_2/n_2 = 55 \times 10/105 = 5.24$

Total $= a_1 d_1/n_1 + a_2 d_2/n_2 = 3.73 + 5.24 = 8.97$

$b_1 c_1/n_1 = 55 \times 10 / 105 = 3.58$

$b_2 c_2/n_2 = 18 \times 22/105 = 3.77$

Total $= b_1 c_1/n_1 + b_2 c_2/n_2 = 3.58 + 3.77 = 7.35$

$$OR_{MH} = \frac{\sum_i^k = a_i d_i / n_i}{\sum_i^k = b_i c_i / n_i} = 8.97/7.35 = 1.22$$

CHAPTER 4

Study Design

Case

Case definition, in epidemiology, set of criteria used in making a decision about an individual who has a disease or outcome event of interest. Establishing a case definition is an important step in quantifying the magnitude of disease in a population.

A Case definition in epidemiology study may be defined as a set of standard criteria for diagnosing a particular disease or health-related problem, by specifying clinical criteria and limitations on person, place and time factor.

A case definition must be clear, simple, and concise, must be very easy to apply for all the individual subjects who have been selected from the population of interest. It typically includes both clinical and laboratory characteristics, which are ascertained by one or many methods like diagnosis by a physician, completion of a survey, or routine population screening methods (Sensitivities and Specificities). Individuals meeting a case definition can be categorized as "confirmed," "probable," or "suspected."

Control

The control can be defined as a reduction in the incidence, prevalence, morbidity or mortality of disease to a locally acceptable level;

Elimination: Elimination of disease is to make zero of the incidence

Eradication: Eradication of disease as permanent reduction of disease in the society.

Whereas the proposed definition of inherent in the definitions of control and elimination is the need for continued intervention measures to prevent re-emergence and re-establishment of transmission. It is needed for continued intervention after reaching control or elimination targets that has been the source of confusion among public health workers, health policy-makers and the politicians who provide resources for infectious disease control. At times, misunderstanding has led to neglect or complete cessation of intervention activities, with concurrent decrease in financial resources, and thus to re-emergence of the target disease.

Case-control Study

The case-control study design is often used in the study of rare diseases or as a preliminary study where little is known about the association between the risk factor and disease of interest.

The case – control study will be used to detect number of subjects with disease under study, then they are considered as case and number of subjects without disease can be considered as control. Both the groups are taken from same population.

In case of case-control study, here the investigator select the subjects with a particular disease, latter they will try to find out the cause and effect relationship between the outcome event and exposed variable. Then ODD ratio can computed using the equation mentioned below to verify whether the exposure variable is harmful or beneficial or neither harmful nor beneficial

$$OR = \frac{\dfrac{P\left(\dfrac{exposed}{disease}\right)}{P\left(\dfrac{unexposed}{disease}\right)}}{\dfrac{P\left(\dfrac{exposed}{disease}\right)}{P\dfrac{unexposed}{disease}}} = \frac{a/c}{b/d} = \frac{a \times d}{b \times c}$$

Cohort-study

Cohort studies are a type of medical research used to investigate the causes of disease, establishing links between risk factors and health outcomes. Cohort studies are usually forward-looking - that is, they are "prospective" studies, or planned in advance and carried out over a period of time.

Cohort studies evaluate a possible association between exposure and outcome by following a group of exposed individuals or subjects over a period of time (often years) to see whether they develop the disease or outcome of interest.

In a nutshell, in Retrospective Cohort Study, all the events - exposure, latent period, and subsequent outcome (ex. development of disease) have already occurred in the past. We merely collect the data now, and establish the risk of developing a disease if exposed to a particular risk factor.

A prospective cohort study is one in which a group of subjects are followed over a period of time to see effect of exposure and what disease/outcome data will be collected to compute relative risk.

Computation of Risk Ratio (Relative Risk)

$$Risk\ ratio = \frac{P(outcome\ /\ exposed)}{P(outcome\ /\ not\ exposed)}$$

$$RR_{MH} = \frac{\sum_{i}^{k} = \left(a_i \left(c_i + d_i\right)/n_i\right)}{\sum_{i}^{k} = \left(c_i \left(a_i + b_i\right)/n_i\right)}$$

Cross-sectional Study

In medical research and social science, a cross-sectional study (also known as a cross-sectional analysis, transversal study, prevalence study) is a type of observational study that analyzes data collected from a population, or a representative subset, at a specific point in time, that is, cross-sectional data.

The research design refers to the overall strategy that you choose to integrate the different components of the study in a coherent and logical way, thereby, ensuring you will effectively address the research problem; it constitutes the blueprint for the collection, measurement, and analysis of data.

Prevalence ratio

$$PR = \frac{P(outcome\,/\,exposed)}{P(outcome\,/\,not\ exposed)}$$

These ratios can have values between 0 to ∞. The value greater than 1 indicates there is a positive association between the exposure and outcome variable. If the value is less than 1 indicates that there is no association between exposure and outcome variables and also indicates negative association between exposure and outcome variables.

Excess Risk

To explain about the absolute measure of the impact of exposure on risk, here the investigator uses the excess risk, which is written as ER and it is obtained using the mathematical equation ER $= P(D/E) - P(D/\overline{E})$

To measure the ER, the same risk components, which are considered in relative risk and odds ratio. The excess risk always lies between -1 and $+1$.

If ER $= 0$, then it indicates that $P(D/E) = P(D/\overline{E})$, that is both D and E are independent.

If ER > 0, this implies that, there is a greater risk of the disease D, when subjects are exposed to risk factor E.

Example: The data listed in the table provides the information about the number of infant mortality of case-control study of mothers Martial status and by birth weight. The Married group is taken as (Control) and not married as (Case). Compute the excessive risk the marital status and low birth weight.

Infant Mortality	Marital Status	
	Married	Unmarried
Death	1000 (a)	800 (b)
Live at 1 year	2500(c)	1000 (d)

Solution:

Infant Mortality	Marital Status		Total
	Married	**Unmarried**	
Death	1000 (a)	800 (b)	1800 (a + b)
Live at 1 year	2500(c)	1000 (d)	3500 (c + d)
Total	3500 (a + c)	1800 (b + d)	N=a + b + c + d= 5300

$$ER = P(D/E) - P(D/\overline{E}) = (800/1800) - (1000/3500)$$
$$= 0.44 - 0.29 = 0.15$$

Attributable Risk

Attributable risk (AR) is the difference in incidence rates of diseases (or death) between the exposed and non-exposed group. It is also called as risk difference to attributable risk.

Generally the attributable risk is a measure of association designed to provide an answer to this question and defined as fraction of all cases of D in the population that can be attributed to E.

It can be obtained by the equation $AR = \dfrac{P(D/E) - P(D/\overline{E})}{P(D/E)}$

$$= \frac{\text{Incidence of disease rate among exposed} - \text{Incidence of disease among non - exposed}}{\text{Incidence of disease rate among expose}}$$

Attributable risk indicates to what extent the disease under study can be attributed to the exposure.

Example: Data about the cigarette smoking and lung cancer is as listed below. Compute attributable risk and explain what is the indication of AR.

Cigarette Smoking	Disease Status	
	Lung Cancer	**No Lung Cancer**
Yes	70 (a)	6930 (b)
NO	3(c)	2997 (d)

Solution:

Cigarette Smoking	Disease Status		Total
	Lung Cancer	**No Lung Cancer**	
Yes	70 (a)	6930 (b)	7000 (a + b)
NO	3(c)	2997 (d)	3000 (c + d)
Total	73(a + c)	9927 (b + d)	N = a + b + c + d = 10000

$$P(D/E) = (70/7000) \times 1000 = 10/1000$$

$$P(D/\overline{E}) = (3/3000) \times 1000 = 1/1000$$

$$AR = ((10 - 1)/10) \times 100 = 90\%$$

90% of the lung cancer among smoker was due to the habit of smoking.

This indicates disease can be reduced, if the factor under studies are controlled. The attributable risk is often used as a measure of how many of disease cases are in the table, while evaluating the importance of prevention program designed to reduce exposure E. Generally AR conceptually assumes a perfect intervention that will eradicate exposure to E.

Second Method for the Computation of Attributable Risk

The disease D in the population, can be explained due the presence of the risk factor E. This can answered by Attributable risk. The attributable Risk is a measure of association and it is designed to provide an answer to the question and defined as the fraction of all cases of D in the population that can be attributed to E. In general the attributable risk can be defined as

$$AR = \frac{P(D) - P(D/\overline{E})}{P(D)}$$

But
$$P(D) = P(D|E)P(E) + P(D|\overline{E})P(\overline{E})$$

$$AR = \frac{P(D/E)P(E) + P(D/\overline{E})P(\overline{E}) - P(D/\overline{E})}{P(D)}$$

$$AR = \frac{P(D/E)P(E) + P(D/\overline{E})P(\overline{E}) - 1)}{P(D)}$$

$$AR = \frac{P(D/E)P(E) - P(D/\overline{E})P(E)}{P(D)}$$

$$AR = \frac{P(E)(P(D/E) - P(D/\overline{E}))}{P(D/E)P(E) + P(D/\overline{E})P(\overline{E})}$$

$$AR = \frac{P(E)[RR - 1]}{P(E)RR + P(\overline{E})}$$

$$AR = \frac{P(E)[RR - 1]}{1 + P(E)(RR - 1)}$$

The above expression clears that the attributable Risk depends on both the strength of association between D and E and the prevalence of the risk factor E.

Example: Compute attributable risk to measure the association between women's with smoking habit (risk Factor) and infant mortality (Outcome or Event) for the data listed in the table.

	Women with Smoking Habit	
Infant Mortality	Smoking	No Smoking
Death	15000	17000
Live at 1 year	1123562	2875341

	Women's Smoking Habit (Exposure)		
Infant Mortality	Smoking	No Smoking	Total
Death	15000	17000	32000
Live at 1 year	1123562	2875341	3998903
Total	1138562	2892341	4030903

P(D)	32000/4030903	0.0079
$P(D/\bar{E})$	17000/2892341	0.0059
AR	$(P(D) - P(D/\bar{E}))/P(D)$	0.26
P(E)	1138562/4030903	0.2825
RR	(15000/1138562)/(17000/2892341)	2.24
AR	P(E)[RR-1]/1+P(E)(RR-1)	0.26

Confidence Interval

The data from a Case – Control study may be summarized in a 2×2 – table is as listed below

Exposure	Disease Status	
	Case	Control
Exposed	a	b
Not Exposed	c	d

(i)   The odds that a case was exposed is
odd's of Cases = a/b and

(ii)   The odd's that a control was exposed is
Odd's for control = c/d

Then the ODD's for the sample selected is OR = $\dfrac{a/b}{c/d} = \dfrac{ad}{bc}$

The confidence can be obtained using the value of variance and the variance can be obtained by the equation

$$\text{Var(ln(OR))} = \frac{1}{a} + \frac{1}{b} + \frac{1}{c} + \frac{1}{d}$$

Here ln is the natural logarithm with base e,. The base e is used, because distribution of risk factor will be in the form of exponential.

Then the approximate 95% confidence interval on the log scale for the given ODD's ratio can be the equation

$$\ln(ad/bc) \pm 1.96 \times \sqrt{\frac{1}{a} + \frac{1}{b} + \frac{1}{c} + \frac{1}{d}}$$

A 95% confidence interval for ODD's ratio under investigation is obtained by exponentiating the two end points

$$\ln(ad/bc) - 1.96 \times \sqrt{\frac{1}{a} + \frac{1}{b} + \frac{1}{c} + \frac{1}{d}}$$

and $$\ln(ad/bc) + 1.96 \times \sqrt{\frac{1}{a} + \frac{1}{b} + \frac{1}{c} + \frac{1}{d}}$$

Example: The role of smoking in pancreatitis has been recognized and data is listed as below. Obtain the confidence interval on the log scale.

Exposure	Pancreatic	
	Case	Control
Current Smokers	38	81
Ex.-smoker	13	80
Never Smoker	2	50

Solution: The ODD's ratio between never smoker and Ex-smoker is

$$\text{OR} = (ad/bc) = (13 \times 50/2 \times 80) = 4.06$$

Then Confidence interval is

$$\ln(ad/bc) - 1.96 \times \sqrt{\frac{1}{a} + \frac{1}{b} + \frac{1}{c} + \frac{1}{d}}$$

$$= \ln(4.06) - 1.96 \times \sqrt{\frac{1}{38} + \frac{1}{81} + \frac{1}{13} + \frac{1}{80}} = -0.128$$

and $$\ln(ad/bc) + 1.96 \times \sqrt{\frac{1}{a} + \frac{1}{b} + \frac{1}{c} + \frac{1}{d}}$$

$$= \ln(4.06) + 1.96 \times \sqrt{\frac{1}{38} + \frac{1}{81} + \frac{1}{13} + \frac{1}{80}} = 2.932$$

Then the confidence interval after taking exponential is $(e^{-0.128}, e^{2.932}) = (0.88, 18.76)$
Similarly Confidence Interval between the current smoker and never smoker is (3.04,56.70)

Confidence Interval of Relative Risk

Example: Estimate the Relative Risk and   95% level confidence interval of relative for the data which is collected by an investigator after conducting a cohort study is as listed in the table.

		Liver Cancer	
		Cases	Controls
Alcohol(Liter per Day)	≥ 1	178	1411
	0	79	1486

Solution:

		Liver Cancer		
		Cases	Controls	Total
Alcohol Drinking status (Liter per Day)	≥ 1	178	1411	1589
	0	79	1486	1565
	Total	257	2897	3154

RR	a/(a+b)/c/(c+d)	2.22
ln(RR)	ln(a/(a+b)/c/(c+d))	0.797
Var(ln(RR))	b/a(a+b) + d/c(c+d)	0.017

95% Confidence Interval	
ln(RR) ± 1.96 × Sqrt(Var(ln(RR))	
ln(RR) - 1.96 × Sqrt(Var(ln(RR))= 0.542	ln(RR) + 1.96 × Sqrt(Var(ln(RR))= 1.053

Take exponential for both the values, then LI = exp(0.542) = 1.72 and UL = 2.87
CI = (1.72,2.87)

Example: Estimate the Relative Risk and   95% level confidence interval of relative risk for the follow-up group of population – based study data as listed in the table.

	Lung Cancer	
	Yes	No
Yes	1200	400
No	300	3100

Solution:

		Lung Cancer		
		Yes	**No**	**Total**
Smoker	Yes	1200	400	1600
	No	300	3100	3400
	Total	1500	3500	5000

RR	a/(a+b)/c/(c+d)	8.50
ln(RR)	Ln(a/(a+b)/c/(c+d))	2.140
Var(ln(RR))	b/a(a+b) + d/C(c+d)	0.003

Randomization

Randomization as a method of experimental control has been extensively used in human clinical trials and other biological experiments. It prevents the selection bias and insures against the accidental bias. It produces the comparable groups and eliminates the source of bias in treatment assignments.

In some early clinical trials, randomization was performed by constructing two balanced groups of patients and then randomly assigning the two groups to the two treatment groups. Most clinical trials today invoke a procedure in which individual patients, upon entering the study, are randomized to treatment.

Randomized Controlled Trial

A randomized controlled trial (or randomized control trial; RCT) is a type of scientific (often medical) experiment which aims to reduce bias when testing a new treatment. The people participating in the trial are randomly allocated to either the group receiving the treatment under investigation or to a group receiving standard treatment (or placebo treatment) as the control.

Randomization minimizes selection bias and the different comparison groups allow the researchers to determine any effects of the treatment when compared with the no treatment (control) group, while other variables are kept constant.

The RCT is often considered as a gold standard for a clinical trial. After randomization, the two (or more) groups of subjects are followed in exactly the same way and the only differences between them is the care they receive.

For example, in terms of procedures, tests, outpatient visits, and follow-up calls, should be those intrinsic to the treatments being compared.

The main goal of randomized trials is therefore to assure that each individual has an equal probability to be assigned to one or the other treatment.

Strengths and Weaknesses of RCTs

Strengths

1. Only type of study able to establish causation
2. Ability to assign and administer treatment or intervention in a precise, controlled way.
3. Decreases selection bias and minimizes confounding due to unequal distribution in a chosen population
4. Measurements can be chosen precisely making it easier to make observations consistently (specially for parametric data)
5. Blinding is easier improving credibility

Bias

The systematic error that will be done in the design or in the conduct of study. This systematic error may happen due to improper selection of study subjects or by not applying proper procedure for gathering relevant exposure and/ or disease information. This may be the root cause for error in result.

The systematic error (bias) needs to be differentiated from error due to random variability (sampling error), which results from the use of a population sample to estimate the study parameters in the reference of population. This sample estimates may differ substantially from the true parameters because of random error.

Bias may exist when on the average, the result of an hypothetically infinite number of studies (related to specific association and reference population) differ from the true results.

The prevention and control of bias can be done in three levels.

1. Ensuring that the study design is appropriate for addressing the study hypothesis
2. Adopting and carefully monitoring the result produced which is required for collection of data, that are very much valid and more reliable.
3. Applying proper analytical technique to analyze the data.

Selection Bias

Selection bias may occurs when a systematic error happens in selecting study subject for case-control study (case-group and Control group) and exposed and unexposed subjects in cohort studies – may lead to distorting the measure expressing the association exposure and outcome.

Information Bias

Information bias is epidemiologic studies results due to imperfect definitions of study variables.

This error may occur due to misclassification of exposure and/ or outcome status for significant proportion of study participants.

The valid study is solid study, like valid claim is solid claim. The valid study will be similar to a unbiased study, when the study is based on its design, methods and procedures.

The exposure identification bias may affect cohort, because in this study is usually ascertained before the outcome (disease) of interest occurs.

Definition: The effect produced by the contrasting actions of two (or more) chemical groups.

Example: **Antagonistic** effect is the effect between the opposing actions of insulin and glucagon to blood sugar level. While insulin lowers blood sugar glucagon raises it.

Definition of synergism: Interaction of discrete agencies (such as industrial firms), agents (such as drugs), or conditions such that the total effect is greater than the sum of the individual effects.

Antagonistic interaction means that the effect of two chemicals is actually less than the sum of the effect of the two drugs taken independently of each other.

An undesirable example of synergism seen in the body is taking depressant drugs and drinking alcohol.

Epidemiological studies have revealed about many risk factors which are root cause for getting major events or diseases like cancer, CVD etc. The common example one consider is association between the lung cancer and cigarette smoking as risk factor.

In the present scenario the investigators focus is towards the interaction of one factor C with the exposure E, on the outcome event D.

When the risk factors C and E are considered as binary levels, then the probability of getting disease can be written as

$$P_{11} = P(D/E\&C), \ P_{10} = P(D/E\&\overline{C}), \ P_{01} = P(D/\overline{E}\&C) \text{ and } P_{00} = P(D/\overline{E}\&\overline{C}).$$

Then the definition of relative risk can be defined by considering neither E nor C as a base line or reference group.

$$RR_{11} = \frac{P_{11}}{P_{00}}, \ RR_{10} = \frac{P_{10}}{P_{00}}, \ RR_{01} = \frac{P_{01}}{P_{00}}$$

Similarly we define OR_{11}, OR_{10}, OR_{01} and ER_{11}, ER_{10} and ER_{01}

To calculate the RR using the OR, consider a single binary exposure scenario:

$$R_1 = \frac{O_1}{1+O_1}$$

$$R_0 = \frac{O_0}{1+O_0}$$

Then the relative risk $\ RR = \dfrac{R_1}{R_0} = \dfrac{\dfrac{O_1}{1+O_1}}{\dfrac{O_0}{1+O_0}} = \dfrac{O_1(1+O_0)}{O_0(1+O_1)}$

This can be extended for two binary exposure variable scenario then

$$RR_{11} = \frac{OR_{11}(1+O_{00})}{(1+O_{11})}$$

$$RR_{10} = \frac{OR_{10}(1+O_{00})}{(1+O_{10})}$$

$$RR_{01} = \frac{OR_{01}(1+O_{00})}{(1+O_{01})}$$

$$OR_{10} = \frac{p_{10}/(1-p_{10})}{p_{00}/(1-p_{00})}$$

$$OR_{01} = \frac{p_{01}/(1-p_{01})}{p_{00}/(1-p_{00})}$$

$$OR_{11} = \frac{p_{11}/(1-p_{11})}{p_{00}/(1-p_{00})}$$

Multiplicative Interaction

When there is interaction in terms of the ratio measure of association, we call this as multiplicative interaction.

When we consider the relative risk, it measures the effect of a factor, when we take R_{10}, it explain the effect of E separate from C. Similarly R_{01} explains the effect of C is separate from E and R_{11} explain the total effect of E and C together. When an investigator consider the $RR_{11} = RR_{10} \times RR_{01}$. This indicates that E and C do not interact multiplicatively

When the equation is considered $RR_{11} = RR_{10} \times RR_{01}$ (or for a rare disease from a case-control study), then $\dfrac{P_{11}}{P_{00}} = \dfrac{P_{10}}{P_{00}} \times \dfrac{P_{01}}{P_{00}}$

Multiplying both side by $\dfrac{P_{00}}{P_{01}}$, then we then the equation $\dfrac{P_{11}}{P_{01}} = \dfrac{P_{10}}{P_{00}}$

Left hand side ratio explains RR for D-E relationship among individuals, who will have characteristics C.

Right hand side ratio explains RR for D-E relationship among individuals, who will not have characteristics C

Additive Interaction

When there is interaction in terms of the difference measure of association or the risk difference, we call it an additive interaction

OR

The additive interaction means, the effect of two chemicals or risk factors is equal to the sum of the effect of the two chemicals or risk factors taken separately. This is happening due to the two chemicals acting on the body via same mechanism.

Example: Effect of aspirin and Motrin, Alcohol and Depression and Tranquilizer and Pain killer

Here we can use the relative risk and add deviation of RR from the null value 1 in order to asses synergism.

This indicates E and C do not interact additively if

$$((RR_{11} - 1) = (RR_{10} - 1) + (RR_{01} - 1) \qquad\qquad .....(4.1)$$

This is equivalent to $(P_{11} - P_{00}) = (P_{10} - P_{00}) + (P_{01} - P_{00})$. This equation is obtained by substituting the values $RR_{11} = \dfrac{P_{11}}{P_{00}}$, $RR_{10} = \dfrac{P_{10}}{P_{00}}$, $RR_{01} = \dfrac{P_{01}}{P_{00}}$. Then we get $RR_{11} - 1 = \dfrac{P_{11}}{P_{00}} - 1$,

$$RR_{10} - 1 = \dfrac{P_{10}}{P_{00}} - 1 \quad RR_{01} = \dfrac{P_{01}}{P_{00}} - 1 .$$

Simplifying these values we get

$$(P_{11} - P_{00}) = (P_{10} - P_{00}) + (P_{01} - P_{00}).$$

This gives the equation $E_{11} = E_{10} + E_{01}$

Example: If $RR_{11} = 50$, $RR_{10} = 10$ and $RR_{01} = 5$, then $RR_{11} - 1 = 50 - 1 = 49, RR_{10} - 1 = 10 - 1 = 9$ and $RR_{01} - 1 = 5, - 1 = 4$.

Substitute these values in the equation $((RR_{11} - 1) = 50 - 1 = 49$

$$(RR_{01} - 1) + (RR_{01} - 1) = 9 + 4 = 13,$$

This indicates that there is an additive interaction, synergistically, with regard to the effect of E and C.

CHAPTER 5

Tests of Association between Exposure and Outcome

Logarithmic and Exponential Functions in Epidemiological Study

Several analytic procedures in epidemiology use exponential and logarithmic functions. Logarithms are closely related to exponential functions. Consider that $y = a^x$ is equivalent to $\log_a(y) = x$, where $\log_a(y)$ is the base a logarithm of y; the number of times we multiply a to get y is equal to x.

For example, how many 2s do we multiply to get 16?

The answer is $2 \times 2 \times 2 \times 2 = 16$, so the logarithm is 4, written as $\log_2 16 = 4$. In other words, log base 2 of 16 is 4. Different base values can be used, but the most common are 10 and e (i.e., 2.71828…). Logarithms of base 10 are called as common logarithms.

Logarithms of base e are called natural logarithms. Base 10 is used more frequently in the fields of engineering and chemistry.

Base e is used in calculus because it is easily integrated and differentiated. Mathematical answers come out naturally (hence the term "natural log," abbreviated as ln), as opposed to requiring additional coefficients when base 10 is used.

In fact, most epidemics bacteria grow approximately exponentially during the initial phase of an epidemic.

Exponential functions have the form $f(x) = b^x$, where $b > 0$ and $b \neq 1$. An example of an exponential function is the growth of bacteria. Some bacteria double every hour. If you start with 1 bacteria and it doubles every hour, you will have 2^x bacteria after x hours. This can be written as $f(x) = 2^x$.

Exponential functions are used to design populations model which are used in epidemiological study, here we will discuss two of the most common applications, they are Population growth, exponential decay,

Straight Line

If a straight line makes an angle θ with the positive direction of the X–axis then tan θ is called as slope or gradient of the straight line. The angle 'θ' is called the inclination of the line to the X-axis. The angle θ is measured from the positive direction of the X–axis in the anticlockwise direction as shown in the figure 5.1.

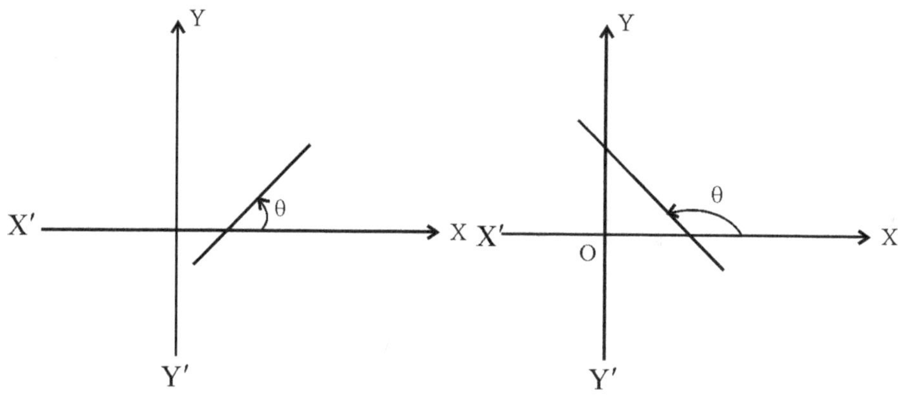

Fig. 5.1

For example, if a straight line makes an angle $45°$ with the positive direction of the X–axis, its slope is tan $45°$ or equal to 1. If a straight line makes an angle $120°$ with the positive direction of x – axis then its slope is tan $120° = \tan(180° – 60°) = – \tan 60° = -\sqrt{3}$.

Slope of a Line Joining Two Points

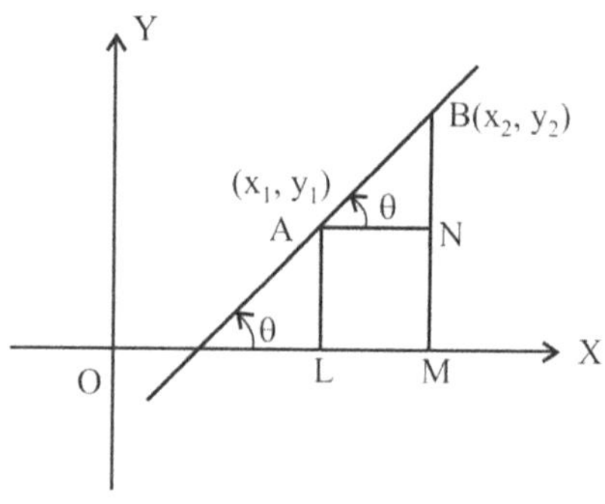

Let A and B be the points (x_1, y_1) and (x_2, y_2) respectively. Let AB be inclined at an angle θ to the x-axis. Draw AL, BM $\perp$ to X-axis and AN $\perp$ to BM. OL $= x_1$, AL $= y_1$, OM $= x_2$, BM $= y_2$

Since AN is $\parallel$ to x-axis, $B\hat{A}N = \theta$

The slope of AB z $= \tan \theta$

$$= \frac{AN}{AB} = \frac{BM-NM}{LM} = \frac{BM-AL}{OM-OL} = \frac{y_2-y_1}{x_2-x_1}$$

$\therefore$ The slope of the line joining the two points (x_1, y_1) and (x_2, y_2) is $\dfrac{y_2-y_1}{x_2-x_1}$

For example, if A $\equiv (3, –4)$ and B$\equiv (–1, 5)$ the slope of $AB = \dfrac{y_2-y_1}{x_2-x_1} = \dfrac{5-(-4)}{-1-3} = \dfrac{9}{-4} = -\dfrac{9}{4}$

Intercepts on x and y axes

In figure if a straight line cuts the x-axis at A and Y-axis at B, OA is called the X-intercept and OB is called the y-intercept of the line. Here in Fig. 5.2(a), both intercepts OA, OB are positive. In Fig. 5.2(b), x-intercept is negative and y-intercept is positive. In Fig. 5.2(c) both intercepts are negative and in Fig. 5.2(d), x-intercept is positive and Y-intercept is negative.

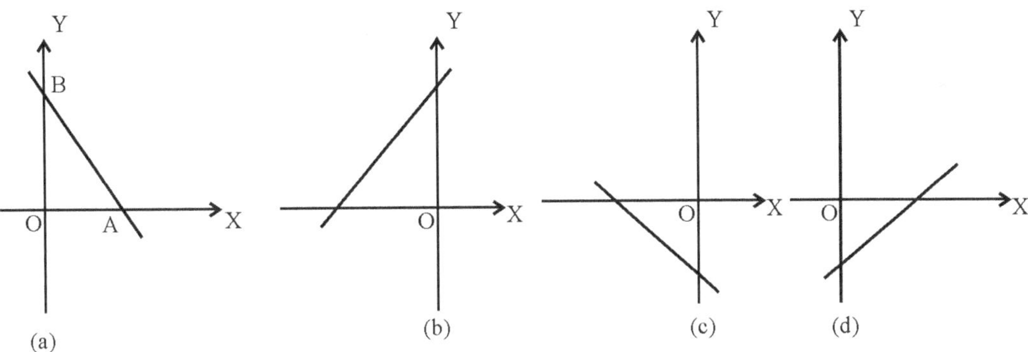

(a) (b) (c) (d)

Fig. 5.2

Equation of a Straight Line Passing through Two Points

Let the straight line pass through the points $A(x_1, y_1)$ an $B(x_2, y_2)$. Let $P(x, y)$ be any point on the line AB.

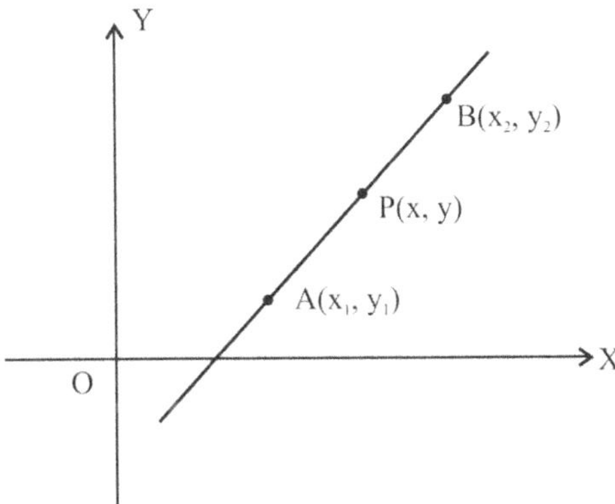

Fig. 5.3

Slope of $AP = \dfrac{y - y_1}{x - x_1}$; Slope of $AB = \dfrac{y_2 - y_1}{x_2 - x_1}$

Since A, P, B lie on the same line, slope of AP = slope of AB

i.e.,
$$\frac{y - y_1}{x - x_1} = \frac{y_2 - y_1}{x_2 - x_1}$$

Hence the equation of the line passing through the points (x_1, y_1) and (x_2, y_2) is

$$\frac{y - y_1}{x - x_1} = \frac{y_2 - y_1}{x_2 - x_1}$$

$$(y - y_1) = \left(\frac{y_2 - y_1}{x_2 - x_1}\right)(x - x_1)$$

Important Properties of Logarithms and Straight Line

1. In logistic regression, the outcome variable is transformed using the natural log, $\ln(p/(1-p))$. If the outcome variable in epidemiology takes on the values 1 or 0, with probability p and $1 - p$, respectively, then the outcome variable does not satisfy certain assumptions used in regression analysis.

2. Poisson regression analysis is appropriate for studying rare diseases in large populations. In Poisson regression, the outcome variable is transformed using the natural log, $\ln(\text{rate})$.

3. Confidence intervals for common epidemiologic measures of association, such as odds ratio, risk ratio, rate ratio, and prevalence ratio.

4. Logarithms are used in both nuclear and internal medicine. For example, they are used for investigating pH concentrations, determining amounts of radioactive decay, as well as amounts of bacterial growth. Similarly exponent function is used to measure the concentration drug distributes in body after every interval of time.

5. Logarithms also are used in obstetrics. When a woman becomes pregnant, she produces a hormone known as human chorionic gonadotropin. Since the levels of this hormone increase exponentially, and at different rates with each woman, logarithms can be used to determine when pregnancy occurred and to predict fetus growth.

6. When an investigator administers particular drug to a patient, the concentration of the drug substance in the body distributes or jumps to the highest level immediately. Then the concentration subsequently decays exponentially. If the doctor or the investigator considers $C(t)$ to represent the concentration at time t, and $C(0)$ to represent the concentration just immediately after the dose is administered then our exponential decay can be written in the exponential model as $C(t) = C(0)\, e^{-kt}$. But the problem that is faced by the physicians is the fact that in most of drugs, where the concentration will be below m, then the drug will be considered as ineffective and a concentration above upper limit M, then the treatment will be considered as dangerous. Thus the physician would like to have the concentration $C(t)$ would lie between $m < C(t) < M$. This means that the initial dose must not produce a concentration larger than M and that another dose will have to be administered before the concentration reaches m. Here logarithm ln (natural log) will be applied reduce that exponential model into regression model and predict the concentration for different intervals of time.

7. The slope between two points will be used to obtain the two parameters a-intercept and b-slope of logistic regression model.

8. LAPLACE TRANSFORM- Pharmacokinetics analysis

The Laplace is one mathematician who developed some mathematical models which are designed to solve engineering problem and the same models can be used Pharmaco-epidemiology studies (Pharmacokinetics analysis) to analyze the distribution, absorption, metabolism, and excretion or elimination drug substances from body.

Pharmaco- epidemiology includes contributions from both these fields, exploring the effects achieved by administering a drug regimen.

The Laplace transform is defined as

***Definition*:** Let f(t) be a function of real variable '*t*' defined for t ≥ 0. Laplace transform of f(t) is denoted by L[f(t)] and is defined by.

$$L[f(t)] = \int_0^\infty e^{-st} f(t) dt$$

Provided the integral on right hand side exists, where s is a parameter real or complex number. The operator L is called the Laplace transform operator.

Clearly, the L[f(t)] is a function of the parameter s. we shall denote this function by F(s).

Thus

$$L[f(t)] = \int_0^\infty e^{-st} f(t) dt = F(s)$$

If F(s) is the Laplace transform of f(t), then f(t) is called the inverse Laplace transform of F(s) and is denoted by $L^{-1}[F(s)]$.

Thus if $\qquad\qquad$ L [f(t)] = F(s)

Then $\qquad\qquad$ f(t) = L^{-1}[F(s)]

The most commonly Laplace transform functions or mathematical equation in Pharmacokinetic studies is $L\left[e^{kt}\right] = \dfrac{1}{s-k}$

and it is derived by applying the definition of Laplace transform

Laplace transform of e^{kt}

By definition

$$= \int_0^\infty e^{-(s-k)t} dt$$

$$= \left[\frac{-e^{-(s-k)}}{s-k} \right]_0^\infty$$

$$= 0 + \frac{1}{s-k} \qquad\qquad [\text{if } s - k > 0]$$

$$\therefore \qquad L\left[e^{kt}\right] = \frac{1}{s-k} \qquad\qquad \text{provided } s - k > 0$$

Inverse Laplace Transform

We have seen that if,

$$L[f(t)] = F(s), \quad \text{then } L^{-1}[F(s)] = f(t)$$

The L^{-1} denotes the inverse Laplace transform.

	F(t)	L[f(t)] = F(s)	F(s)	$L^{-1}[F(s)] = f(t)$
1	1	$\dfrac{1}{s}$	$\dfrac{1}{s}$	1
2.	t^n	$\dfrac{n!}{s^{n+1}}$	$\dfrac{1}{s^n}$	$\dfrac{t^{n-1}}{(n-1)!}$
	e^{kt}	$\dfrac{1}{s-k}$	$\dfrac{1}{s-k}$	e^{kt}

These Models can also be used many processes that take place in the interaction between an organism and a chemical substance. The commonly model in Pharmacokinetic analysis is, the multi-compartmental model is the most commonly used approximations to reality; however, the complexity involved in adding parameters with that modeling approach means that mono-compartmental models and above all two compartmental models are the most-frequently used.

The mathematical model divides this pharmacokinetic model into various compartment, which are named as ADME (Absorption, distribution, Metabolism and Excretion or elimination). These are main processes which are involved in pharmacokinetics and Pharaco-epidemiology.

Commonly it is referred as LADME when the liberation is included as a separate step from absorption.

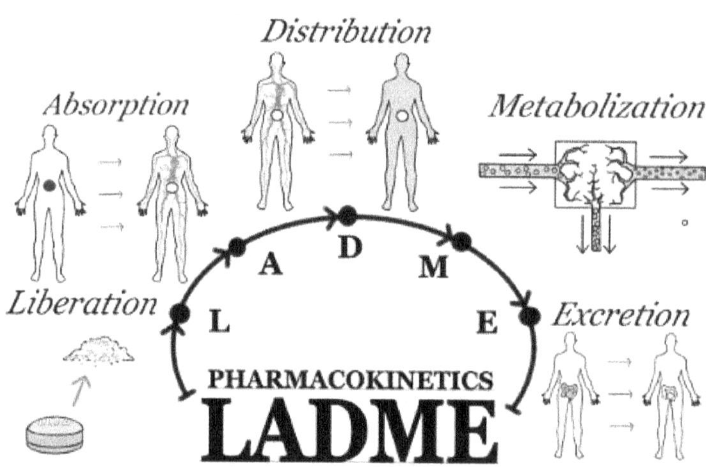

L - Liberation – the process of release of a drug from the pharmaceutical formulation.

A - Absorption – the process of a substance entering the blood circulation.

D - Distribution – the dispersion or dissemination of substances throughout the fluids and tissues of the body.

M - Metabolism (or biotransformation, or inactivation) – the recognition by the organism that a foreign substance is present and the irreversible transformation of parent compounds into daughter metabolites.

E - Excretion – the removal of the substances from the body. In rare cases, some drugs irreversibly accumulate in body tissue

Laplace Transform of Derivative

The Laplace transform of derivative is a technique that can be applied in Pharmaco-epidemiology to convert the differential equation of drug concentration into Laplace transform to design Pharmacokinetics models.

We shall express the Laplace transform of the derivative of a function in terms of the function itself. This property of Laplace transform is very useful, as the operation of differentiation may be replaced by simple algebraic operation of the Laplace transforms.

Definition: A continuous functions f(t) for t > 0 is said to be of exponential order if

$$\lim_{t \to \infty} e^{-st} f(t) = 0$$

***Theorem* 1**: Let *f (t)* be of exponential order and have *f' (t)* which is continuous.

If $\qquad\qquad L[f(t)] = F(s)$

Then $\qquad\qquad L[f'(t)] = sF(s) - f(0)$

Proof: By definition, we have

$$L[f'(t)] = \int_{0}^{\infty} e^{-st} f'(t)\, dt$$

$$L[f'(t)] = \left[e^{-st} f(t) \right]_{0}^{\infty} + s \int_{0}^{\infty} e^{-st} f(t)\, dt$$

[Integration by parts]

$$= 0 - f(0) + s\, L[f(t)]$$

[Because f(t) is of exponential order]

$\therefore \qquad\qquad L[f'(t)] = s\, L[f(t)] - f(0)$

or $\qquad\qquad L[f'(t)] = s\, F(s) - f(0)$

The above result can be extended to 2nd order derivatives.

Corollary: $L[f''(t)] = s^2 F(s) - f(0) - f'(0)$

Proof: Consider

$$F[f''(t)] = L\{[f'(t)]'\}$$

$$= sL[f'(t)] - f'(0) \qquad \text{[By theorem 1]}$$

$$= s\{sL[f(t)] - f(0)\} - f'(0)$$

$$= s^2 L[f(t)] - sf(0) - f'(0)$$

$$= s^2 F(s) - sf(0) - f'(0)$$

or $\qquad L[f''(t)] = s^2 F(s) - s^2 F(s) - sf(0) - f'(0)$

In general, we have

$$L[f^{n}(t)] = s^n F(s) - s^{n-1} f(0) - s^{n-2} f'(0) \dots - f^{n-1}(0),$$

Pharmacokinetic One-compartment Model

One of the most common and the useful route of drug administration is the oral route, where the dosage forms (drug products) such as tablets, capsules, or oral solutions are generally used is one-Compartmental model. In this case we can develop pharmacokinetic models to explain and predict the disposition of drug substances kinetically. After using this model when it is possible to predict by a pharmacokinetic model, then dosing regimens for an individual patient or groups of patients can be calculated using that mathematical model.

The one-compartment open model is the simplest way to describe the process of drug distribution and elimination in the body. This model assumes that the drug can enter or leave the body (i.e., the model is "open"), and the entire body acts like a single, uniform compartment.

IV Bolus - Linear One Compartment Model

In this case the elimination drug substance is expressed by a single first order process by the rate constants as Ke and elimination takes place as shown in the Fig. 5.4.

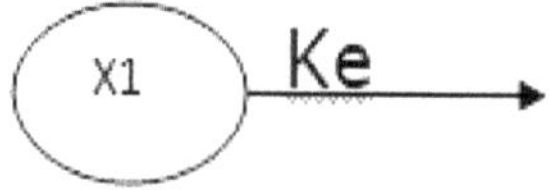

Fig. 5.4

Then the linear one compartment model with one elimination process can be written in the form of differential equation for the rate of change of X1 as

$$\frac{dX1}{dt} = -KeX1 \qquad \qquad .....(5.1)$$

Next step we have to transform this first differential equation into Laplace transform by applying the technique transforming derivative to Laplace transform. The equation obtained after transforming is written as

$$S\overline{X1} - X1(0) = -Ke\overline{X1} \qquad \qquad .....(5.2)$$

After rearranging the terms in the equation 5.2 , we get

$$\overline{X1}\ (s + Ke) = X1(0) \qquad \qquad .....(5.3)$$

At the when time t is 0, then X1(0) is considered as Dose and X1(0) in the equation should be replaced by Dose

$$\overline{X1}\ (s + Ke) = Dose$$

$$\overline{X1} = \frac{Dose}{(s + Ke)}$$

Take Laplace transform both side, then the final to compute concentration of drug

$$X1 = Dose \times e^{-Ket} \qquad\qquad .....(5.4)$$

Here e represents the base of the natural logarithms

After taking the logarithm both sides of the equation 5 we get

$$Ln(x1) = ln(Dose \times e^{-ket})$$
$$Ln(X1) = Ln(Dose) + Ln(e^{-ket})$$
$$Ln(X1) = Ln(Dose) +(-kt)$$
$$Ln(X1) = Ln(Dose) - kt$$

After converting this equation into common logarithm (base is 10), then we get

$$Log(X1) = log(Dose) - \frac{kt}{2.303}$$

Intravenous Infusion - One Compartment Model

When drug is administered intravenously at a constant rate, then the rate of change in drug in body with respect to time can be obtained by the differential equation.

$$\frac{dX}{dt} = k_0 - kX \qquad\qquad .....(5.5)$$

Here K_0 is considered as rate of drug infusion and K is elimination rate constant

After applying the technique of Laplace to derivative, we get

$$S\overline{X} = \frac{k_0}{S} - K\overline{X}$$

Rearrange the terms $\quad S\overline{X} + K\overline{X} = \frac{k_0}{S}$

$$\overline{X}(S+K) = \frac{k_0}{S}$$

$$\overline{X} = \frac{k_0}{S(S+K)}$$

To calculate total amount of drug in the body, the equation $\dfrac{K_0}{S(S+K)}$ has to be resolved into

partial fraction form

$$\frac{K_0}{S(S+K)} = \frac{A}{S} + \frac{B}{S+K}$$

Take LCM

$$\frac{1}{S(S+K)} = \frac{A(S+K)+B(S)}{S(S+K)}$$

$$1 = A(S+K) + B.S \qquad \qquad \qquad .....(5.6)$$

Put $S = 0$ in (5.6)

$$1 = A(0+K) + B.0$$

$$1 = A.K$$

$$A = \frac{1}{k}$$

Put $\qquad\qquad S + K = 0 \rightarrow S = -K$

Substitute $S = -K$ in equation (5.6)

$$1 = A\,(S+K) + B.S$$

$$1 = A.0 + B(-K)$$

$$B = -\frac{1}{K}$$

$$\frac{K_0}{S(S+K)} = \frac{A}{S} + \frac{B}{S+K}$$

$$\frac{1}{S(S+K)} = \frac{A}{S} + \frac{B}{(S+K)}$$

$$\overline{X} = \frac{k_0}{S(S+K)}$$

$$\overline{X} = \frac{K_0}{K_S} - \frac{K_0}{K(S+K)}$$

Take inverse Laplace transform both side, then we get

$$X = \frac{K_0}{K} - \frac{K_0}{K}e^{-kt}$$

$$X = \frac{K_0}{K}(1 - e^{-kt})$$

If X is replaced by concentration C then the equation can be written as

$$C = \frac{K_0}{K}(1 - e^{-kt})$$

Pharmacokinetic Two-compartment Model in Pharmaco-Epidemiology Study

In case of two compartment model the body will be divided into *central* and *peripheral* compartment. The first compartment consists of Plasma and tissues and the second compartment consists of tissues, where slow distribution of drugs takes place inside the body.

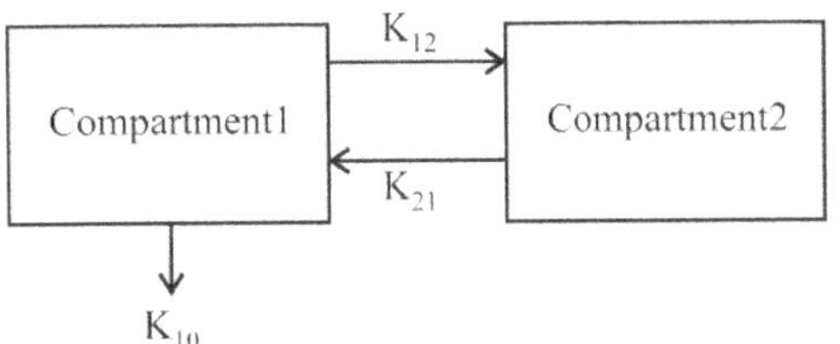

In a two compartment model the amount of drug in each compartment is taken as X_1 and X_2, the micro rate constants describing drug transfer between or out of the compartment (Ks) is expressed by the differential equations as

$$\frac{dX_1}{dt} = k_{12}X_2 - k_{21}X_1 - k_{01}$$

$$\frac{dX_2}{dt} = k_{21}X_1 - k_{12}X_2$$

Apply Laplace transform both side of the differential equations

$$L\left\{\frac{dX_1}{dt}\right\} = L\left\{k_{12}X_2\right\} - L\left\{k_{21}X_1 + k_{10}X_1\right\} \qquad .....(5.7)$$

$$L\left\{\frac{dX_2}{dt}\right\} = L\left\{k_{21}X_1\right\} - L\left\{k_{12}X_2\right\} \qquad .....(5.8)$$

$$S\overline{X1} - \overline{X1}(0) = k_{12}\overline{X2} - (k_{21} + k_{10})\overline{X1}$$

$$(S + k_{21} + k_{10})\overline{X1} - \overline{X1}(0) = k_{12}\overline{X2}$$

$$S\overline{X2} - \overline{X2}(0) = k_{21}\overline{X1} - k_{12}\overline{X2}$$

Because of normalization $\overline{X}1(0) = 1$ in central compartment

$$(S + k_{21} + k_{10})\overline{X1} - 1 = k_{12}\overline{X2}$$

$$(S + k_{21} + k_{10})\overline{X1} - k_{12}\overline{X2} = 1 \qquad .....(5.9)$$

$$-K_{21}\overline{X1} + (S + K_{12})\overline{X2} = 0 \qquad .....(5.10)$$

These two equations are in the system of linear equations which are solved by the method of Crammer's rule

$$a_1x + b_1Y = c_1$$

$$a_2x + b_2Y = c_2$$

$$\Delta = \begin{pmatrix} a_1 & b_1 \\ a_2 & b_2 \end{pmatrix} = a_1b_2 - a_2b_1$$

$$\Delta_1 = \begin{pmatrix} a_1 & c_1 \\ a_2 & c_2 \end{pmatrix} = a_1c_2 - a_2c_1$$

$$\Delta_2 = \begin{pmatrix} c_1 & b_1 \\ c_2 & b_2 \end{pmatrix} = c_1 b_2 - c_2 b_1$$

$$\Delta = \begin{pmatrix} s + k_{10} + k_{21} & -k_{12} \\ -k_{21} & s + k_{12} \end{pmatrix}$$

$$= (s + k_{10} + k_{21})(s + k_{12}) - (-k_{21} - k_{12})$$

$$= s^2 + (k_{10} + k_{12} + k_{21})s + k_{10}k_{12}$$

Take

$$a + b = (k_{10} + k_{12} + k_{21})$$

$$ab = k_{10}k_{12}$$

$$\Delta = s^2 + (a+b)s + ab$$

This is a quadratic equation

$$\Delta = (s + a)(s + b)$$

$$\Delta_1 = \begin{pmatrix} 1 & -k_{12} \\ 0 & s + k_{12} \end{pmatrix} = 1(s + k_{12}) - 0$$

$$\Delta_1 = s + k_{12}$$

$$\overline{X1} = \frac{s + k_{12}}{(s+a)(s+b)}$$

After finding the partial fraction for above rational function

$$\frac{(s + k_{12})}{(s+a)(s+b)} = \frac{A}{s+a} + \frac{B}{s+b}$$

$$\overline{X1} = \frac{k_{12} - a}{(b-a)(s+a)} + \frac{k_{12} - b}{(a-b)(s+b)}$$

Take Inverse Laplace Transform both side

$$X_1 = \frac{k_{12} - a}{b - a}e^{-at} + \frac{k_{12} - b}{b - a}e^{-bt}$$

$$X_1 = Ae^{-at} + Be^{-bt}$$

Exposure at Several Discrete Levels

Test of Association between Baseline Variable and Several Discrete Variables

This variable is also referred to as the exposure, the explanatory variable, or the independent variable. In a regression model this variable is used to predict or explain the outcome variable or disease.

Suppose exposure variable E has k natural levels, named as 1,2,3 …..k. First level of variable will be taken as baseline variable and with the remaining k-1 level of variable investigator measures the association between exposure level and baseline or reference level.

In this case the null hypothesis H_0 is defined when D and E are considered as independent, the H_0: $RR_2=RR_3=…..RR_k= 1$.

When the OR is considered, then H_0: $OR_2=OR_3=…..=OR_k= 1$. Or $ER_2=ER_3=…..=ER_k= 0$, because RR = OR for the value of $2\leq k\leq K$.

When D and E are not independent, then the investigator defines the alternative hypothesis. Then the alternative hypothesis can be written as $H_A : RR_k\neq 1$

The general form of the table can be written as

		Disease		Total
		DiseaseD	**NO Disease $\overline{D}$**	
	1	a_1	b_1	m_1
	2	a_2	b_2	m_2
Exposure Levels	3	a_3	b_3	m_3
	……..	………	………..	
	……..	………	………	
	K	a_k	b_k	m_k
	Total	nD	$n\overline{D}$	$n= m_1+m_2+…m_k$

The chi-Square test can be allied to compute the test value and degree of freedom can be taken as k-1.

The mathematical equation that will be used to compute test value is

$$\chi^2= \frac{n^2}{nD\,n\overline{D}}\sum_{i=1}^{K}\frac{\left(a_i - \dfrac{ndm_i}{n}\right)}{m_i}$$

***Example* 1:** The data given in the table is about the survey done by an investigator about the different category of people based on the number of cigarette they take per day and attack of lung cancer is listed below. Verify the level of association between the incidence of lung cancer due to smoking habit.

		Disease		Total
		Disease D	**No Disease $\overline{D}$**	
Number of cigarette a	0	12	60	72
subject smoke per day	1-2	120	270	390
(Smoking)	3-4	105	150	255
	≥ 5	80	120	200
	Total	317	600	917

Solution:

Computation of Predicted or Expected Values

A_i	$A_i = (nd \times m_i)/n$	$A_i = (nd \times m_i)/n$
A_1	(317×72)/917	24.89
A_2	(317×390)/917	134.8201
A_3	(317×255)/917	88.15158
A_4	(317×200)/917	69.1385

a	A	$(a-A)^2$	$(a-A)^2/mi$
12	24.89	166.15	2.31
120	134.82	219.63	0.56
105	88.15	283.87	1.11
80	69.14	117.97	0.59
			$\Sigma(a-A)^2/m_i = 4.574$
test	20.2		

Test value $= \lambda^2 = 20.2$

Degree of freedom $\lambda = (r-1)(c-1)$

$= (4-1)(2-1)$

$= 3$

$P = 0.00015$

The difference is significant and there is a strong association between smoking habit and lung cancer

Example 2: The data given in the table is about the survey done by an investigator about the different category of people based on the body weight and heart attack is listed below. Verify the level of association between the incidence of heart problem due to more weight.

		Disease		Total
		Heart attack D	No heart attack $\overline{D}$	
Body weight (Kg)	50-60	25	90	115
	60-70	150	260	410
	70-80	110	150	260
	≥ 80	80	135	215
	Total	365	635	1000

Solution:

Computation of Predicted or Expected Values

A_i	$A_i=(nd \times m_i)/n$	$A_i=(nd \times m_i)/n$
A_1	$(365 \times 115)/1000$	41.98
A_2	$(365 \times 410)/1000$	149.65
A_3	$(365 \times 260)/1000$	94.9
A_4	$(365 \times 215)/1000$	78.475

a	A	$(a-A)^2$	$(a-A)^2/m_i$
25	41.98	288.3204	2.507134
150	149.65	0.1225	0.000299
110	94.90	228.01	0.876962
80	78.475	2.325625	0.010817
			$\sum(a-A)^2/m_i =3.395$
test	14.6		
P	0.0021		

$$\lambda^2 = \frac{n^2}{nD\, n\overline{D}} \sum_{i=1}^{K} \frac{\left(a_i - \dfrac{ndmi}{n}\right)}{mi}$$

$$\lambda^2 = 14.6$$

Degree of freedom $\quad \lambda = (r-1)(c-1)$

$$- (4-1)(2-1) = 3$$

$$P = 0.0021$$

The difference is significant and there is a strong association between body weight and heart attack.

Test for Trend in Risk

Two Scientist Cochran and Armitage introduced or derived a method to test for trend to measure the association between the outcome event D and risk factor that is exposed at different levels. As the exposure level is increased and each levels of exposures are quantified. In many of epidemiological study the exposure, the measurement scale not only possess a natural ordering, but also associated with the numerical scale. This is possible when the investigator considers the risk factor like age, body weight and risk factors like tobacco consumption and alcohol drinking etc.

In this situation investigator focus on the alternative to null hypothesis of independence, say H_1 : $RR_2 < RR_3 < \text{--------} < RR_k$ or $RR_2 > RR_3 > \text{--------} > RR_k$. In case when relative risks of all exposure levels are same, then the Null hypothesis will be considered. Then $H_0 : RR_2 = RR_3 = \text{----------} = RR_k = 1$.

For each level of exposure, there will be a numerical value x_k. The test trend value $P(D/E = x_k)$ against scaled exposure x_k can be drawn on the graph sheet and that will be based on exposure level x_k. Then the statistical test value can be computed to verify or to give an evidence suggesting that trend value is increasing or decreasing as exposure level decreases.

For quantitative variable, here the investigator will assign the value 0, 1, 2, 3------ to the different categories of exposure and then apply test statistics to verify the effect of exposure using the equation.

$$\lambda^2_{trend} = \frac{n^3}{nD\,n\overline{D}} \frac{\left[\sum_{i=x}^{k} k\left(a_k - \frac{nd\,m_k}{n}\right)\right]^2}{\left[\sum_{i=1}^{k} x_k^2 m_k - \left(\sum_{i=1}^{k} x_k m_k\right)^2\right]}$$

Example: The data given in the table is about the survey done by an investigator about the different category of people based on the body weight and coronary heart disease as listed below. Verify the level of association between the incidence CHD problem due to more weight of different level.

		Coronary Heart Disease		Total
		CHD D	NO CHD $\overline{D}$	
Body	≤ 60	35	550	
weight	60-70	50	510	
(Kg)	70-80	70	560	
	80-90	85	495	
	≥ 90	90	600	

Solution:

		Coronary Heart Disease		Total
		CHD D	NO CHD $\overline{D}$	
	≤ 60	35	550	585
Body weight	60-70	50	510	560
(Kg)	70-80	70	560	630
	80-90	85	495	580
	≥ 90	90	600	690
	Total	nD =330	$n\overline{D}$ = 2715	n =3045

Expected Values codes	Equation to compute expected value	Expected values of Diseased Group
A_0	(330×585)/3045	63.4
A_1	(330×560)/3045	60.69
A_2	(330×630)/3045	68.28
A_3	(330×580)/3045	62.86
A_4	(330×690)/3045	74.78

Category No.(x_k)	a_i	A_i	$(a_i - A_i)$	$X_{i(a_i - A_i)}$
0	35	63.4	−28.4	$0 \times (-28.4) = 0$
1	50	60.69	−10.69	$1 \times -10.69 = -10.69$
2	70	68.28	1.72	$2 \times 1.72 = 3.44$
3	85	68.6	22.14	$3 \times 22.14 = 66.42$
4	90	74.78	15.22	$4 \times 15.22 = 60.88$
				$\sum_{i=x_{i(a_i-A_i)}}^{k} = 120.05$
				$\left[\sum_{i=x_{i(a_i-A_i)}}^{k} \right]^2 = 14412$

$$n^3 = (3045)^3 = 18947900$$

$$n^3 \times \left[\sum_{i=x_k(a_k-A_i)}^{k} \right]^2 = 4.06899E+14$$

$$nD / n\overline{D} \times \left[n\sum_{i=1}^{k} x_k^2 m_k - \left(\sum_{i=1}^{k} x_k m_k \right)^2 \right] = 1.6976E+13$$

$$\lambda_{trend}^2 = \frac{n^3}{nD\, n\overline{D}} \frac{\left[\sum_{i=x}^{k} k\left(a_k - \frac{nd\, m_k}{n} \right) \right]^2}{\left[\sum_{i=1}^{k} x_k^2 m_k - \left(\sum_{i=1}^{k} x_k m_k \right)^2 \right]}$$

$$\lambda_{trend}^2 = 23.97$$

Degree of freedom = (2 − 1) = 1

P = 0.00009

Graphs 1

Construction of Scattered graph between Body weight category and Probability of getting disease due to different category of body weight.

Body Weight	P(D/E)
1	0.185
2	0.361
3	0.408
4	0.404

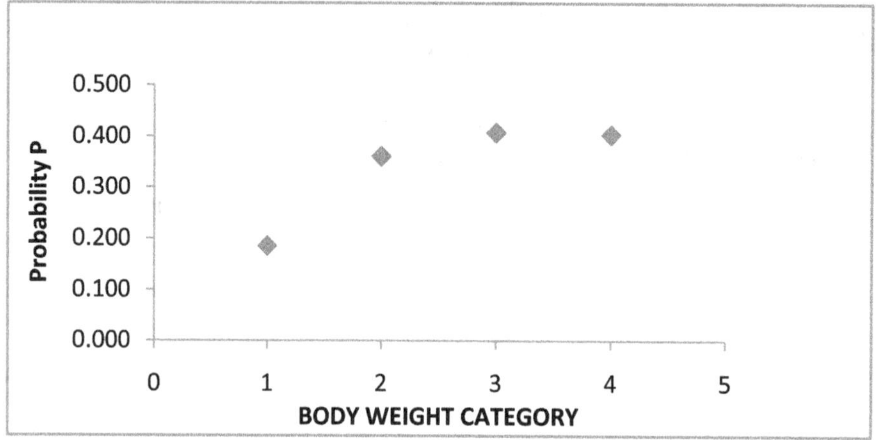

Graphs 2

Construction of Scattered graph between Body weight category and Odds Ratio of getting disease due to different category of body weight.

Body Weight	(P/1P)
1	0.23
2	0.56
3	0.69
4	0.68

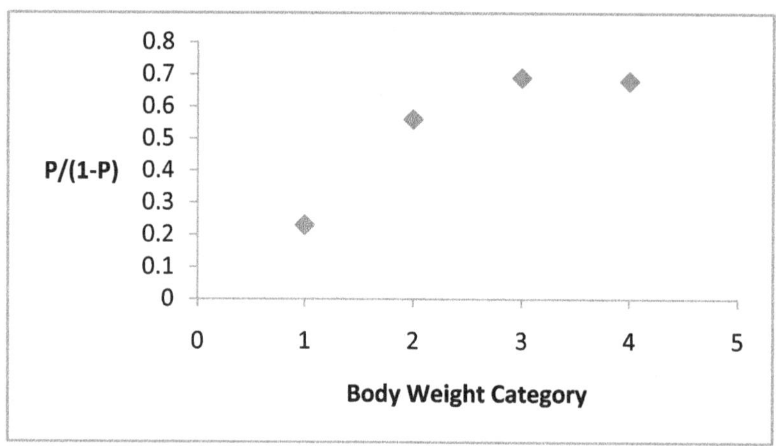

Graphs 3

Construction of Scattered graph between Body weight category and Odds Ratio of getting disease due to different category of body weight.

Body Weight	LOG(P/1-P)
1	−1.47
2	−0.58
3	−0.37
4	−0.39

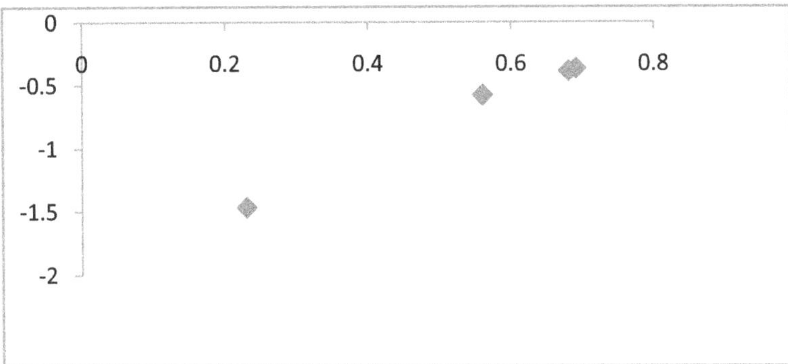

Kaplan – Meier Survival Estimate

This function estimates survival rates and hazard from data that may be incomplete. Here we introduce the product limit (PL) method for estimating the survival rates, it is also called as Kaplan-Meier method. The interval for survival time will be taken as [0, T].

This is a non-parametric statistic used to estimate the survival function from lifetime data. In medical research, it is often used to measure the fraction of patients living for a certain amount of time after treatment

Let $t_1 < t_2 < \ldots\ldots < t_k$ be the different times of deaths of the sample of size n which is chosen from a homogeneous population and the survival function s(t) can be estimated for $k \leq n$, the k could be less than n, because some subjects may be censored and some subjects may have events at the same time.

Let n be the number of subjects at risk at the time just prior to t_i ($1 \leq i \leq k$). Then the survival function can be obtained by the equation $\hat{S}(t) = \pi_{t_i < t}^{k}\left(1 - \dfrac{d_i}{n_i}\right)$.

It is named as product limit estimator or Kaplan-Meier estimator where t_i is duration of study at point i, d_i is number of deaths up to point i and n_i is number of individuals at risk just prior to t_i. S is based upon the probability that an individual survives at the end of a time interval, on the condition that the individual was present at the start of the time interval. S is the product (P) of these conditional probabilities.

The 95% confidence interval can be obtained by the equation $\hat{S}(t)$ is $\pm \exp(1.96\ \hat{S}(t)$ and the variance $\hat{S}^2(t) = \Sigma_{ti<t} \dfrac{d_i}{n_i(n_i - d_i)}$

An important advantage of the Kaplan–Meier curve is that this method can take into account some types of censored data, particularly right-censoring, which occurs if a patient withdraws from a study, is lost to follow-up, or is alive without event occurrence at last follow-up. On the plot, small vertical tick-marks indicate individual patients whose survival times have been right-censored. When no truncation or censoring occurs, the Kaplan–Meier curve is the complement of the empirical distribution function.

Example:

t_i	n_i	d_i	$1-d_i/n_i$	$S(t_i)$
7	22	3	0.8636	0.8636
9	19	1	0.9474	0.8182
11	15	1	0.9333	0.7636
13	12	1	0.9167	0.7000
16	10	1	0.9000	0.6300
22	7	1	0.8571	0.5400
23	6	1	0.8333	0.4500

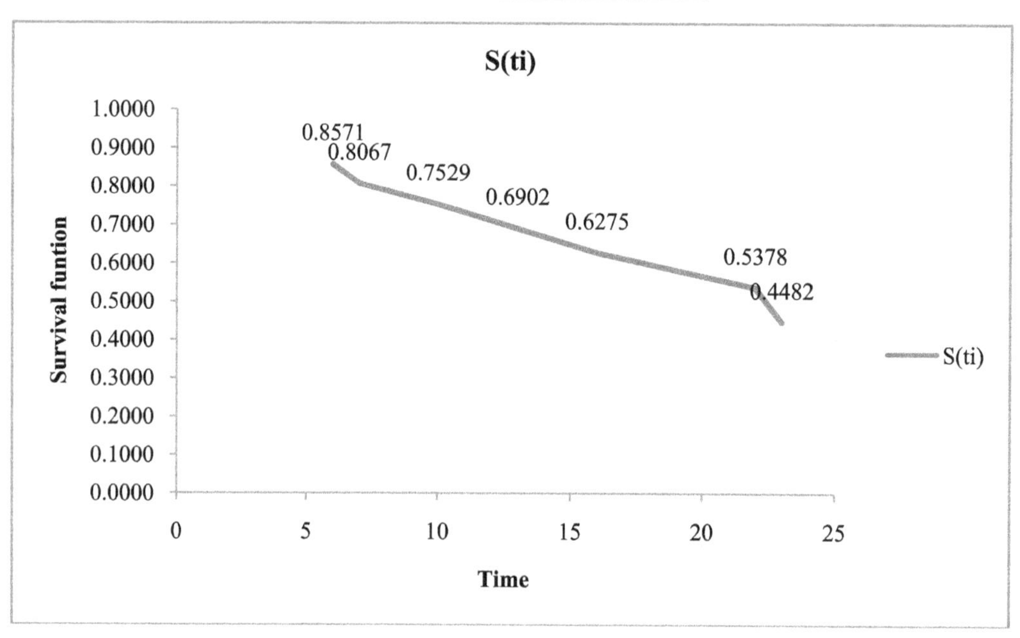

Mathematical Equation to Compute Survival Function

Compute survival function we need to compute probability of death, which depends upon the number of deaths and mid year population (p_x) for each year age (x) of a particular calendar year. Here investigator need to calculate q_0, which is obtained by the equation $q_0 = \dfrac{D_0(1-f)}{B^t} + \dfrac{D_0(f)}{B^{t-1}}$, here D_0 is taken as the number of deaths of infants, B^t is the number of births in the year t and B^{t-1} is number of births in the year t-1. Here the investigator assumes that lx, the number of survivors at the age x, declines linearly between the time t and t + 1 and occurred between x to x + 1 is equal to $x + \dfrac{1}{2}$. Latter l_x is obtained by the equation $l_x = L_x + \dfrac{1}{2} d_x$, L_x Persons lived between the years x and x+ 1. Then the value of qx is computed usin the equation $= \dfrac{dx}{L_x + \dfrac{1}{2}dx}$. The simplified for this equation is $\dfrac{R_x}{1+\dfrac{1}{2}R_x}, R_x = \dfrac{dx}{L_x}$. This is a conditional probability of death between the x and x +1.

$d_x = l_x - l_{x+1}$, number of deaths between the year interval x to x+1.

p_x =Probability of surviving between the year interval x to x + 1.

$L_t = l_{t-1} - (1 - q_{t-1})$ = Number alive at the beginning of the interval. L_0 = the is an arbitrary value, in general that will be taken as 100000.

$d_t = l_t - l_{t+1} = q_t \times l_t$ = number of deaths during the time interval t to t + n

$p_t = (1 - q_t)$ – Probability of surviving in the time interval

$S(t) = \dfrac{l_t}{l_0}$ = Proportional at the time t, that have not yet failed, cumulative probability of surviving at the beginning of the time interval or at the end of the previous interval

$$S(t+1) = p_{(t+1)} \times S(t)$$

After performing the Censoring

Wt = number Censored during the interval

$l^1 = l_t - \dfrac{wt}{2}$ = adjusted number at risk of the event in the interval

$$q_t = \dfrac{d_t}{1 - l_t^i}$$

Life Table

Age Interval Column	Probability of dying during the time interval	Number alive at the beginning of the time	Number of deaths during the time interval	Cumulative Survival
00-01	0.02592	100000	2592	100000
01-05	0.0042	97408	409	0.97408
5-10	0.00232	96999	225	0.9958
10-15	0.00202	96774	195	0.99768
15-20	0.00443	96579	428	0.99798
20-25	0.0061	96151	587	0.99557
25-30	0.00632	95564	604	0.9939
30-35	0.00654	94960	621	0.99368
35-40	0.01098	94339	1036	0.99346
40-45	0.01765	93303	1647	0.98902
45-50	0.02765	91656	2534	0.98235
50-55	0.04387	89122	3910	0.97235
55-60	0.05987	85212	5102	0.95613
60-65	0.09654	80111	7734	0.94014
65-70	0.13654	72377	9882	0.90346
70-75	0.18765	62494	11727	0.86345
75-80	0.2544	50767	12915	0.81235
80-85	0.37886	37853	14341	0.74562
85-90	0.47897	23511	11261	0.62111
90-95	0.5791	12250	7094	0.52103
95+	1	5156	5156	0.4209

The Column 1 consists of age interval, x to x+n: Age interval between exact ages for each row of the life table.

The Column 2 the proportional values q_x of the population in each age interval that are alive at the beginning of the interval, and dead before reaching the end of the interval. The proportion is computed from the observed mortality rates of an actual population and is used to derive the remaining columns of the table.

The Column 3 represents the number of persons alive at the beginning of the age interval and it is denoted as l_x

The values mentioned in **Column 4** denotes the number of persons dying during the age interval and denoted as d_x

When a person dies or enters the next higher age interval, their place is immediately taken by someone entering from the next lower age interval. The number of persons in the age interval remains the same.

The values in the L_x and T_x columns are based on the assumption that an additional 100,000 persons are added to the table annually and are subject to the mortality rates computed in the column4. The population is considered stationary because the total population and the number of people in each age interval do not change.

The **Column 5** represents cumulative survival function S(t), which is obtained by the equation

$$S(t) = \frac{l_t}{l_0}$$

Fisher Exact Test

It is known that Chi-Square test is a approximate test. The approximation is inadequate when sample sizes are small, or the data are very unequally distributed among the cells of the table, resulting in the cell counts predicted on the null hypothesis (the "expected values") being low. The usual rule of thumb for deciding whether the chi-squared approximation is good enough is that the chi-squared test is not suitable when the expected values in any of the cells of a contingency table are below 5, or below 10 when there is only one degree of freedom. Under the assumption that row and column totals or marginal totals are fixed.

In this method we use probability theory to obtain the probability of observed table, taking the fixed marginal totals. Here the table will be written as

Risk Factor Status	Disease Status		Total
	Disease	No Disease	
Exposed	a	b	a +b
Not Exposed	c	d	c +d
Total	a + c	b + d	N=a + b + c + d

With the probability of observed outcomes a,b,c,d and marginal totals (a+c), (b+d), (a+b) and (c+d) which are fixed, then Fisher's exact test is obtained by the equation

$$P = \frac{(a+c)!(b+d)!(a+b)!(c=d)!}{n!a!b!c!d!}$$

Where n! = n(n – 1)(n – 2)............3.2.1

Example: The data given below, is about the Hypertension status of pregnant women with twins of the sample or subjects taken from the population of particular country. Compute Fishers Exact for the data listed in the table.

Risk Factor	Hypertension Status		Total
	Yes	No	
Best Rest	2	50	52
Normal Rest	6	42	48
Total	12	106	N=100

$$P = \frac{(a+c)!(b+d)!(a+b)!(c+d)!}{n!a!b!c!d!}$$

$$P = \frac{(12)!(106)!(52)!(48)!}{100!2!50!6!42!}$$

$$= 0.09$$

In general, if the Chi-Square, continuity-Corrected Chi-square and Fisher's tests give different inferences, then Fisher exact test should be used.

Binomial Distribution

The Binomial distribution is one of the most widely encountered probability distribution which is used in statistics. Binomial distribution is also known as "Bernoulli distribution" after the Swiss mathematician James Bernoulli (1654 – 1705) who discovered in the year 1700 and the same was published in the year 1713.

The Binomial distribution used under the condition that when:

(i) The random experiment is performed repeatedly in a finite and fixed number of time. Here we consider n is finite and fixed number of trials.

(ii) The outcome of the random experiment (trial) results will be obtained in dichotomous classification of events. The events are classified as success (the occurrence of the event) and failure (the non occurrence of the event).

(iii) If p is the probability of success for one trial and q = 1 - p, is the probability of failure and that will be constant for each trial.

(iv) Trails are independent of one another in that probabilities associated with the outcomes in one trial are not influenced by the outcomes in another trial

Definition: If P is probability of success and q is probability of failure for one trial. If N is total number of trial (repeated N-times), X- is number of success in N-trial. Then N-X is total number of failure, then $P(X) = {}^{N}C_{X}p^{X} q^{(N-X)}$

This equation can also be written with a particular condition as $P(X=r/n, p) = {}^{N}C_{X}p^{X} q^{(N-X)}$

Where   p= Probability of success for one trial

1-p = probability of failure for one trial

N = number of trials

X = number of success

Here the investigator mainly focus on computing the probability of the random variable when the number of success is X, that takes the value r, that is, the probability of success occurs exactly r times in N trials for the chance p (Success for one trial).

Example: When certain drug is known to cause some side effect of 10% at certain time and if five patients are treated with that drug, what is probability that 4 or more may get side effect. If treating of 5 patients repeated 30 times, compute the probability of having 7 or more of 30 patients having side effects.

Solution:

Let X be the side effect and given that p= 10% = 0.1

Then $q = 1 - p = 1 - 0.1 = 0.9$

But $P(X) = {}^{N}C_{X} p^{X} q^{(N-X)}$

When $X = 4$

$$P(4) = {}^{5}C_{4} (0.1)^{4} (0.9)^{(5-4)}$$

$$= \frac{5\ 4\ 3\ 2}{1\ 2\ 3\ 4} (0.1)4 (0.9)1$$

$$= 5 (0.1)4 (0.9)$$

Similarly

$$P(5) = {}^{5}C_{5} (0.1)^{5} (0.9)^{(5-5)}$$

$$= \frac{5\ 4\ 3\ 2\ 1}{1\ 2\ 3\ 4\ 5} (0.1)^{5} (0.9)^{0}$$

$$= (0.1)^{5}$$

Then the probability of 4 or more is

$$P(4 \text{ or More}) = P(5) + P(4) = (0.1)^{5} + 5 (0.1)^{4} (0.9)$$

$= 0.00046$

Given that n=30 and p = 0.1, then mean = $\mu = np = 30 \times 0.1 = 3$

The standard deviation $\sigma = \sqrt{npq} = \sqrt{30 \times 10 \times 0.9} = 1.64$

There $P(x \geq 7) = P\left(z \geq \left(\frac{x - \mu}{\sigma}\right)\right) = P\left(z \geq \left(\frac{7-3}{1.64}\right)\right) = 0.0075$

The probability of 7 or more of thirty patients having side effect is less than 1%

Poisson Distribution

Poisson distribution was derived in 1837 by a French mathematician Simeon D. Poisson (1781-1840). Poisson distribution may be obtained as limiting case of Binomial probability distribution under the following conditions:

1. n, the number of trials we perform on subjects or animals must be very large or indefinitely large i.e.,

   $n \to \infty$.

2. p, the constant probability of success for each trial becomes very small , it may tend to zero p
   $\to 0$

3. $np = \lambda$ will be finite one

With all the three conditions mentioned above, the Poisson distribution is defined as

$$P(x) = \frac{\lambda^x e^{-\lambda}}{x!}$$

Where e = 2.7183

Generally, Poisson distribution is applicable where there are number of random situations and the probability of a success on a single trial is small and the number of trials is very large.

The Poisson probability distribution can be applied in epidemiological studies to determine the probability of rare events. For example, it can be used obtain the number of cells in a given volume of fluid, or the number of bacterial colonies growing in a certain amount of medium and it also describes the behavior of rare events (with small probabilities) such as patients arriving at an emergency room, decaying radioactive atoms etc. In case of Poisson distribution the mean and variance will be equal to λ (Lambda- Greek letter). The λ is one of the important value, which is required to characterize any Poisson distribution.

It is also used to measure the probability that a certain number of events occur within a certain period of time. The events need to be unrelated to each other and also need to occur with a known average rate

Example: When 1000 corona patients treated and probability of cure is 0.001, then compute the probability of 5 patients cures for n = 1000 and p=0.0001

Solution: $\quad P(X = r/\lambda) = \dfrac{\lambda^x e^{-\lambda}}{x!}$

$$\lambda = np = 1000 \times 0.001 = 1$$

$$P(X = 5/1) = \frac{1^5 e^{-1}}{5!} = 0.0030$$

Normal Distribution

If X is a continuous random variable following normal probability distribution with mean μ, standard deviation σ, then its probability density function is given by the equation.

$$P(x) = \frac{1}{\sigma\sqrt{2\pi}} e^{\frac{-(x-\mu)^2}{2\sigma^2}} \qquad -\infty < x < \infty$$

This equation can also be written as

$$y = \frac{1}{\sigma\sqrt{2\pi}} e^{\frac{-(x-\mu)^2}{2\sigma^2}} \qquad -\infty < x < \infty$$

where $\pi = 3.14$, e = 2.7183 (base of Natural logarithms)

Since the normal measured on a continuous scale, it can be used the measure the probability of continuous variables like height, weight, BP lies within a particular range.

Properties of Normal Distribution

1. The graph of the p(x) is the in the form of bell-shaped curve. The top of the bell is directly above the mean.
2. The normal curve is symmetrical about the mean μ;
3. The mean is at the middle and divides the area into halves.
4. The total area under the curve is equal to 1;
5. It is completely determined by its mean and standard deviation σ (or variance σ^2)
6. No portion of curve lies below the x-axis, since p(x) being the probability can never be negative.
7. Theoretically, the range of the distribution is between $-\infty$ and ∞, practically, Range $= 6\sigma$
8. Near the mean value, the normal curve is concave, while near $\pm 3\ \sigma$, the curve is convex to the horizontal axis. The points of inflection, i.e., the points where the change in curvature occurs are $\pm 1\sigma$;
9. Within a range 0.6745 of the σ on both sides of the mean 50% of the frequencies occur. This is probable error;
10. The area lying between the normal curve and horizontal axis is said to be the area under curve and is equal to the number of frequencies in the distribution. The standard deviation distributes the area under the normal curve as given below.
    (a) Mean $\pm 1\sigma$ covers 68.268% area. 34.134% area will lie on either side of the mean.
    (b) Mean $\pm 2\sigma$ covers 95.725% area. 47.725% area will lie on either side of the mean.
    (c) Mean $\pm 3\sigma$ covers 99.73% area. 49.865% area will lie on either side of the mean. It covers almost all the area, leaving only 0.27% area outside the curve

A graph of this standardized (mean 0 and variance 1) normal curve is shown

Standard Normal Curve showing percentages Mean $\mu = 0$, Standard deviation $\sigma = 1$

This normal distribution can be applied to analyze the problems of epidemiology, because some variables distribute normally. For example, the body mass index tends to distribute normally. Rather than applying the integral calculus to obtain area under the curve to obtain probability density function for specific value, we can apply Normal distribution by transforming the value into Gaussian distribution using population mean μ and standard deviation σ, then for the computed value of Z, area under the curve is obtained using standard normal distribution table.

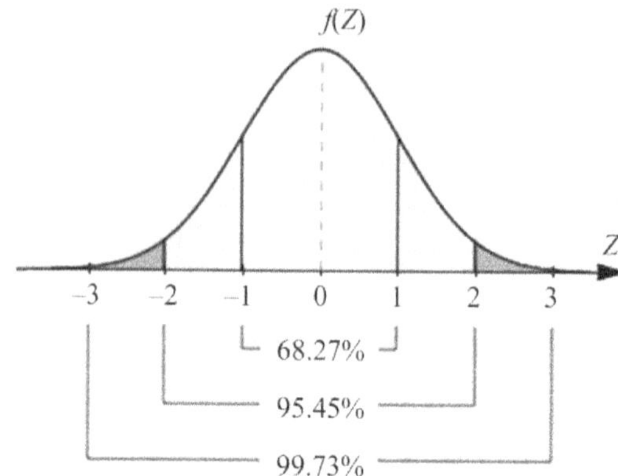

The Gaussian value is obtained by the $Z = \dfrac{x-\mu}{\sigma}$, where x – is a random variable with mean μ and standard deviation σ

Areas Under Standard Normal Curve

Distance from the mean ordinates in terms of ±σ	Area under the curve
Z = ± 0.6745	50% = 0.50
Z = ± 1.00	68.26% = 0.6826
Z = ± 1.96	95% = 0.95
Z = ± 2.00	95.44% = 0.9544
Z = ± 2.58	99% 0.99
Z = ± 3.0	99.73% 0.9973

Example: If the total cholesterol value for a normally distributed population is found to be 200 mg/ 100 ml mean and 20 mg / 100 ml standard deviation. What is the probability that an individual will have cholesterol value? (a) 140 and 200 mg/100 ml

Solution:

Here we have calculate P(180≤x≤200).

To find that, transform both the variables to Z

When x = 140 and μ = 200, $Z = \dfrac{x-\mu}{\sigma}$, $Z = \dfrac{140-200}{20} = -40/20 = -2$

When x = 200 $Z = \dfrac{200-200}{20} = 0$

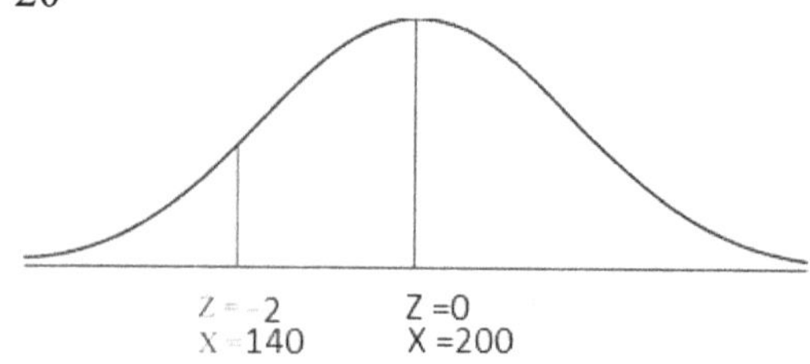

Here we have to calculate area between z = 0 and z = –1

$$P(140 \leq x \leq 200) = P(-2 \leq Z \leq 0) = P(0 \leq Z \leq 21) = 0.4772 = 47.72\%$$

Confounding and Interaction

Generally, in epidemiological study, the investigator considers two variables, termed as risk factor and disease or outcome variable. But in a study, there may be one more variable, that can be called as third factor, which may have an important influence on the risk factor and outcome event disease. If third factor can explain the relationship between Risk factor and outcome event, then that factor is called as confounder. Then the investigator decides the presence of confounder.

Adjusting the confounding variable is achieved by using logistic modeling by fitting the confounder with the risk factors. Comparison of deviations, for the model with confounder model and another model without confounder and risk factor gives the information, whether the risk factor is still important after allowing for the confounder. Then the ODDs ratios are compared, then the effect of confounder can be known. However, we could reasonably conclude no confounding in the study at hand if the odds ratios unadjusted and adjusted, were similar.

If third factor makes some modification in the relationship between Risk factor and Disease, then we can say that there is interaction. Whenever the epidemiological study is designed or analyzed then the issue of confounder and interaction need to consider.

If there are more than one confounder and interactions are identified, then the third factor can be termed as set of factors.

Concept of Confounder

A confounder is an extraneous or irrelevant factor that can have some effect on outcome or event (Disease status) along with the main risk factor. There are two possible cases of confounder.

1. In the first the confounder is the relationship to appear
2. In the second case the confounder is going to hide a true relationship.

For identifying Confounding, compute the measure of association before and after adjusting for a potential confounding factor. If the difference between the two measures of association is 10% or more, then confounding was present. If it is less than 10%, then there was little, if any, confounding.

Characteristics of a confounding variable

General characteristics of confounders are

1. A true confounding factor is predictive of the outcome event in the absence of the exposure.
2. A confounding factor is also associated with the exposure being studied but is not a proxy or surrogate for the exposure.

Potential confounders

A confounder (or 'confounding factor') is something, other than the thing being studied, that could be causing the results seen in a study. Confounders have the potential to change the results of research because they can influence the outcomes that the researchers are measuring.

In Epidemiology a confounder is not part of the real association between exposure and disease, predicts disease and unequally distributed between exposure groups. A researcher can only control a study or analysis for confounders that are known and measurable.

Example: Grey hair predicts heart disease if it is put into a multiple regression model because it is unequally distributed between people who do have heart disease (the elderly) and those who don't (the young). Grey hair confounds thinking about heart disease because it is not a cause of heart disease.

Strategies to reduce confounding: The following are important strategies to reduce confounding effect,

1. Randomization (aim is random distribution of confounders between study groups)
2. Restriction (restrict entry to study of individuals with confounding factors - risks bias in itself)
3. Matching (of individuals or groups, aim for equal distribution of confounders)
4. Stratification (confounders are distributed evenly within each stratum)
5. Adjustment (usually distorted by choice of standard)
6. Multivariate analysis (only works if you can identify and measure the confounders)

Interaction

Generally, the investigator assumes the presence of a single factor, which is considered as a root cause for aetiology of a disease. When more than one factors involved in disease aetiology, then we are going study how the multiple factors interact in causing a disease.

When the incidence rate of disease in the presence of two or more risk factors differs the incidence, rate expected to result from their individual effect. In that situation the investigator can make different strata, then measures the association of exposures and the outcome or event. Here the investigator measures incident without interaction and with interaction of exposures. If the incidence of interaction between two factors greater than the individual factor, then the interaction effect between those factors will be taken into account and they will be considered causative factor getting a particular disease or outcome.

The term interaction is used in epidemiology to describe a situation, in which two or more risk factors modify the effect of each other with regard to the occurrence of event or level of given outcome.

A minimum of three factors are needed for the study of interaction effect and outcome. When we consider Y as outcome variable, Age is considered as main risk factor and third factor (potential effect modifier) is considered as z. To analyze this data we need to compute attributable risk and relative risk.

The interaction terms are named as product terms. This interaction term can also consider in multiple logistic regression model to analyze the data.

Example: In a sample of 600 subjects chosen from a population are, the subjects are stratified into different subgroups on the basis of different factor like age, smoking habit, consumption of alcohol and outcome event (Coronary heart disease). The data is as listed in the below.

Risk Factor (Smoking)		CHD(Yes)	CHD (No) Control
AGE<50	Exposure	35	45
	Non Exposure	10	30
Total			

Risk Factor (Smoking)		CHD(Yes)	CHD (No) Control
AGE -50 -60	Exposure	50	70
	Non Exposure	20	50

Risk Factors (Interaction of Smoking and Consumption of Alcohol)	CHD(Yes) (Case)	CHD (No) (Control)
AGE ≥ 60 Exposure-both	70	120
Non Exposure-both	30	60

Third strata is due to interaction effect of smoking and consumption of alcohol.

Generalized Odds for Ordered (2 x k) – Tables

In this section, we will be able to generalize the concept of odds ordinal outcomes. Here data will be written in two rows and K- columns.

	Columns level						
Rows	1	2	3			K	Total
1	a_1	a_2				a_k	A
2	b_1	b_2				b_k	B
Total	N1	N2				nk	N

Here we can have different generalization by noting that an ODD's ratio can be interpreted as an ODD's for a different events.

Now we present the concept of generalized odds, a special statistics specifically formulated to measure the strength of such trend and will use the same and explain its use.

Here we have to obtain the two values, namely concordances and discordance.

Concordance = $a_1(b_2 + b_3 ---- + b_k) + a_2(b_3 + b_4 + ---- + b_k) + ---------- +_{ak\,-1} b_k.$

Discordance = $b_1(a_2 +- a_3 ---- + a_k) + b_2(a_3 + a_4 + -------- + a_k) + ---- + b_{k-1} a_k$

To measure the degree of association, we calculate the ODD's ratio , it is written as Θ = C/D

The product in number of concordance pairs C (ex $a_1 b_2$) go from upper left corner to lower right corner.

Similarly, the product in the number of discordance pairs D (eg b_1a_2) go from left to upper right. Then the data can be analyzed as per ODD's ratio. This method is most ideal to analyze the association of case-control with an ordinary risk factor.

Example: The data of Case-Control study of the epidemiology of preterm delivery, as listed below. Obtain the ODD's ration

	AGE				
	14-17	18-19	20-24	25-29	≥30
Cases	10	20	45	55	34
Controls	15	26	18	120	80

Solution:

The Concordance = C = 10×(26 + 18 + 120 + 80) + 20(18 + 120 + 80) + 45(120 + 80) + 55(80)

$$= 20200$$

The Discordance = D = 15(20 + 45 + 55 + 34) + 26(45 + 55 + 34) + 18(55 + 34) + 120(34)

$$= 11476$$

$$\Theta = C/D = 20200/11476 = 1.76$$

This implies that the younger mother would be more likely to have a preterm delivery.

Absolute Risk

It is the ratio of people who have a medical event compared to all of the people who could have an event.

AR (absolute risk) = the number of events (good or bad) in treated or control groups, divided by the number of people in that group.

Example: If 30 out of 100 subjects are get dementia in their lifetime, the absolute risk is 30/100 or 30%. The higher the denominator (the bottom number), the lower the absolute risk.

Absolute Risk of Control Group (ARC): It is defined as the absolute risk of events in the control group or Placebo group, and it is denoted as ARC

Absolute Risk of Treatment Group (ART): It is defined as the absolute risk of events in the treatment group or Case group, and it is denoted as ART

ART = the AR of events in the treatment group

ARR (absolute risk reduction) = ARC – ART

The differences between relative and absolute risk reductions are often poorly understood by health professionals, and even more poorly understood by patients. However, these concepts are critical for communicating information to your patients.

The event rate is the proportion of people in the population who experience the particular event. The event rate changes according to baseline risk. While an event rate is reported in a clinical trial, you can only ever estimate an event rate for your patient using an understanding of their disease and risk factors.

The relative risk reduction is the difference in event rates between two groups, expressed as a proportion of the event rate in the untreated group.

For example, if 20% of patients die with treatment A, and 15% die with treatment B, the relative risk reduction is 25%. If the treatment works equally well for those with a 40% risk of dying and those with a 10% risk of dying, the absolute risk reduction remains 25% across all groups.

The absolute risk reduction is the arithmetic difference between the event rates in the two groups. This varies depending on the underlying event rate, becoming smaller when the event rate is low, and larger when the event rate is high. In the example above, there is a 5% absolute risk reduction with treatment B if the event rate is 20%. However, as the event rate increases to 40%, the absolute risk reduction increases to 10%. As the event rate decreases to 10%, the absolute risk reduction decreases to 2.5%. The treatment still works just as well, but the numbers have changed.

If a patient is told that treatment B reduces their risk of dying by 25% (the relative risk reduction), they may make a different decision to the one they would make when told that treatment B reduces their risk of dying by 2.5%.

The number needed to treat is calculated as 1/ARR. It is the number of people that you would have to treat with treatment B in order to save one additional life. In the examples above, treatment B may give a NNT that varies from 10 to 40 depending on the expected event rate.

Definition

The Number Needed to Treat (NNT) is the number of patients you need to treat to prevent one additional bad outcome (death, stroke, etc.). For example, if a drug has an NNT of 5, it means you have to treat 5 people with the drug to prevent one additional bad outcome.

How do you calculate number needed to treat?

Calculation

1. The NNT is the inverse of the absolute risk reduction (ARR).
2. The ARR is the absolute difference in the rates of events between a given activity or treatment relative to a control activity or treatment, ie control event rate (CER) minus the experimental event rate (EER), or ARR = CER - EER.

How do you calculate absolute risk reduction?

How to calculate risk

1. ARC = the AR of events in the control group
2. ART = the AR of events in the treatment group
3. ARR (absolute risk reduction) = ARC – ART.
4. RR (relative risk) = ART / ARC.

Risk terms

AR (absolute risk) = the number of events (good or bad) in treated or control groups, divided by the number of people in that group

ARC = the AR of events in the control group

ART = the AR of events in the treatment group

ARR (absolute risk reduction) = ARC – ART

RR (relative risk) = ART / ARC

RRR (relative risk reduction) = (ARC – ART) / ARC

RRR = 1 – RR

NNT (number needed to treat) = 1 / ARR

Examples

- RR of 0.8 means an RRR of 20% (meaning a 20% reduction in the relative risk of the specified outcome in the treatment group compared with the control group).
- RRR is usually constant across a range of absolute risks. But the ARR is higher and the NNT lower in people with higher absolute risks.
- If a person's AR of stroke, estimated from his age and other risk factors, is 0.25 without treatment but falls to 0.20 with treatment, the ARR is 25% – 20% = 5%. The RRR is (25% – 20%) / 25% = 20%. The NNT is 1 / 0.05 = 20.
- In a person with an AR of stroke of only 0.025 without treatment, the same treatment will still produce a 20% RRR, but treatment will reduce her AR of stroke to 0.020, giving a much smaller ARR of 2.5% – 2% = 0.5%, and an NNT of 200.

Significant difference

- If the RR (the relative risk) or the OR (the odds ratio) = 1, or the CI (the confidence interval) = 1, then there is no significant difference between treatment and control groups.
- If the RR >1, and the CI does not include 1, events are significantly more likely in the treatment than the control group.
- If the RR <1, and the CI does not include 1, events are significantly less likely in the treatment than the control group.

Relative Hazard

The Hazard ratio gives the information about instantaneous risk at a particular time, when the time interval of interest is considered and it will be labeled as [0, T] on the appropriate time scale which is very much relevant for the study which is designed by an investigator. The hazard function, conventionally denoted, is defined as the event rate at time t conditional on survival until time t or later (that is, $T \geq t$). It is the probability density function of the distribution of mortality. Here the investigator can obtain Hazard function incidence rate at exact time t in that particular interval [0, t]. Here the investigator label the Hazard functions into two groups as $h(t)_E$ for exposed group and $h(t)_{\bar{E}}$ (Non-exposed group. The quantitative measure of the relative difference of the incidence between exposed and unexposed group or population can be obtained by the equation

$$RR_t = \frac{I(t)_E}{I(t)_{\overline{E}}}$$ for the interval $[0, t]$. This interval of time is chosen on the fixed interval or the interval which is labeled as $[0, T]$.

Then the relative Hazard between exposure and incidence in non-exposure is obtained using the mathematic equation

$$RR_H = \frac{H(t)_E}{H(t)_{\overline{E}}}$$

The hazard functions considers not only the total number of events, but also consider the timing of each event.

Relative hazard could take any value which varies at different time t's within the labeled interval $[0, T]$. At certain point of time the $RH(t_1) > 1$, this implies that the exposure or risk factor increases the risk of disease D at time t_1.

If $RH(t_2) < 1$ at any other point, implies that the exposure or risk factor decreases the risk of disease D at time t_2.

If $RH(t)$ remains constant over the time interval $[0, T]$ implies the relative impact of exposure on the instantaneous incidence rate remain constant over time.

This Hazard ratio function is used in clinical trial statistics, which helps the investigator or doctor to give a conclusion with confidence saying that healing or recovery of subjects is faster with new drug, when patients were treated with new drug.

Time	Survivors (n_i)	Deaths(e_i)	Interval (u_i)	Hazard (h_t)=e_i/n_iu_i
0	26	0	10	0.0000
10	26	1	2	0.0192
12	25	1	1	0.0400
13	24	1	2	0.0208
15	23	1	1	0.0435
16	22	1	4	0.0114
20	22	3	4	0.0341
24	19	3	2	0.0789
26	16	2	1	0.1250
27	14	1	12	0.0060
39	13	1	3	0.0256
42	12	1	3	0.0278
45	10	2	3	0.0667
48	8	1	4	0.0313
52	7	1	6	0.0238
58	6	1	2	0.0833
60	5	1	1	0.2000
61	4	1	1	0.2500
62	3	1	11	0.0303
73	2	1	2	0.2500
89	2	1	16	0.0313

Baseline Hazard Function

The baseline hazard function, that is not estimated within the model, but is a hazard function obtained when we set all covariate as zero. In many applications, it is very important to have an estimate of the baseline hazard function, or more generally the baseline distribution function.

Assessing Risk Factor

In epidemiology, investigators are very much interested in evaluating the chance that, who is possessing certain attribute, with specific disease. The most common which is used in epidemiology is probability. That measures an individual becoming a newly diseased, say that the individual has the attribute under consideration. That attribute is considered as the risk of disease. This risk measuring is the probability of disease incidence.

Even though risk is a useful summary of the relationship between risk factor and disease, that would be not sufficient for assessing the importance of the risk factor to disease outcome. As in most of the procedures in epidemiological study, a comparison group is required. The group should be like Case (with disease) and Control (Without disease).This helps to give the definition of relative and its application in epidemiological study.

Example: The data listed below gives the result of a cross – section study of peripheral vascular disease (PVD) due to cigarette smoking.

Without Stratification

	PVD		
Cigarette Smoking	**YES**	**NO**	**Total**
YES	20	1700	1720
NO	50	1200	1250
Total	70	2900	2970

With Stratification

	PVD		
Cigarette Smoking	**YES**	**NO**	**Total**
Current Smoker	18	1600	1618
Ex-Smokers	42	1000	1042
Never Smoker	10	600	610
Total	70	2900	2970

Testing Association between Exposure and Outcome Variable

Cochran–Mantel–Haenszel Test

The Cochran–Mantel–Haenszel (CMH) test which is used to measure the strength of the association between an exposure and disease or response, after classifying the data into different strata. The method is used with a dichotomous outcome variable and a dichotomous risk factor. We stratify the data into two or more levels of the confounding factor. In essence, we create a series of two-by-two tables showing the association between the risk factor and outcome at two or more levels of the confounding factor, and we then compute a weighted average of the risk ratios or odds ratios across the strata (i.e., across subgroups or levels of the confounder).

In this method, observed confounders are taken into account for the analysis. Investigator first state a null hypothesis H_0. Here he assumes that D and E are independent, controlling for the possible confounding effect of C and assuming no interaction between C and E.

Hypothesis is stated for various measures of association as

$$H_0 : OR_1 = OR_2 = \ldots\ldots OR_I = 1$$

$$RR_1 = RR_2 = \ldots..RR_I = 1$$

$$ER_1 = ER_2 = \ldots\ldots ER_I = 0$$

The alternative hypothesis H_1 may be considered when D and E are not independent and the investigator assumes at least one of the Odds Ratio will be different from 1, this indicates, there is interaction. Second form of alternative hypothesis is $H_2 : OR_1 = OR_2 = OR_3 = \ldots\ldots OR_I \neq 1$. Here each stratum provides a separate piece of evidence regarding independence of D and E.

Before computing a Cochran-Mantel-Haenszel Estimate, it is important to have a standard layout for the two by two tables for each stratum. The general format of the table is written below

	Outcome Present	Outcome Absent	Total
Risk Factor Present(Exposed)	a	b	a+b
Risk Factor Absent(Unexposed)	c	d	c+d
Total	a+c	b+d	n

Using the notation in this table investigator can compute the risk ratio or an odds ratio as follows

Cochran-Mantel-Haenszel Estimate for a Risk Ratio

$$\hat{RR}_{cmh} = \frac{\sum \dfrac{a_i(c_i + d_i)}{n_i}}{\sum \dfrac{c_i(a_i + b_i)}{n_i}}$$

$$OR_{MH} = \frac{\left(\Sigma\left(a_i d_i / n_i\right)\right)}{\left(\Sigma\left(b_i d_i / n_i\right)\right)}$$

Where a_i, b_i, c_i, and d_i are the numbers of participants in the cells of the two-by-two table in the ith stratum of the confounding variable, and n_i represents the number of participants in the ith stratum.

1. Form different strata i of confounding variables

2. For each stratum obtain predicted frequency of the upper left-hand cell (For the variable a_i, corresponding predicted variable $e_i = ((a_i + b_i) \times (a_i + c_i))/ n_i$

3. v_i–variance for each value ai is obtained using the equation $v_i = (a_i + b_i)(c_i + d_i)(a_i + c_i)(b_i + d_i)/ n_i^2 \times (n_i - 1))$

4. Then the CMH –test statistic λ_{CMH}^2 is computed using the equation

5. $$\lambda_{CMH}^2 = \frac{\left(\sum_{i=1}^{I} a_i - \sum_{i=1}^{I} e_i\right)^2}{\sum_{i=1}^{I} v_i}$$

6. The null hypothesis is rejected and alternative hypothesis is accepted, when there is an association between disease and risk factor. This can be verified when the computed value of test statistics is greater than the tabulated value of Chi-square for the degree of freedom 1for 5% or 1% level of significance.

Example: For the data given below compute the Relative Risk and odd Ratio to measure the association between obesity and CVD and data has been stratified into two categories. One with age <50 and those who were $\geq$ 50 at baseline:

Table of Obesity and Incident Cardiovascular Disease by Age Group

	Age < 50					Age ≥ 50		
	CVD	No CVD	Total			CVD	No CVD	Total
Obese	10	90	100		Obese	36	164	200
Not Obese	35	465	500		Not Obese	25	175	200
Total	45	555	600		Total	61	339	400

Solution:

Age < 50 Years			
	CVD	No CVD	Total
Obese	10	90	100
Not Obese	35	465	500
Total	45	555	600

$$RR = \frac{\dfrac{10}{100}}{\dfrac{35}{500}} = \frac{0.10}{0.07} = 1.43$$

or

$$OR = \frac{\dfrac{a}{b}}{\dfrac{c}{d}} = \frac{ad}{bc} = \frac{10 \times 465}{90 \times 35} = 1.48$$

Age ≥ 50 Years			
	CVD	No CVD	Total
Obese	36	164	200
Not Obese	25	175	200
Total	61	339	400

$$RR = \frac{\dfrac{36}{200}}{\dfrac{25}{400}} = \frac{0.18}{0.125} = 1.44$$

$$OR = \frac{\dfrac{a}{b}}{\dfrac{c}{d}} = \frac{ad}{bc} = \frac{36 \times 175}{25} = 1.54$$

And, using the same data we can compute the **Cochran-Mantel-Haenszel estimate for the odds ratio** as follows

$$OR_{MCH} = \frac{\left(\Sigma(a_i d_i / n_i)\right)}{\left(\Sigma(b_i c_i / n_i)\right)} = \frac{\dfrac{10 \times 465}{600} + \dfrac{36 \times 175}{400}}{\dfrac{90 \times 35}{600} + \dfrac{164 \times 25}{400}} = 1.44$$

Woolf's Method on the Logarithm Scale

Consequently, **Woolf's Method** is based on Weighing each stratum according to its sampling error, giving the most weight to those strata that have the smallest variance. This method uses the simple idea of averaging the individual stratum estimates of the odds Ratio.

In all of our studies, we are just taking a sample of the population and we know there is always the threat of sampling error.

The potential for sampling error is best seen in the variance of the measure of association for each stratum and also **Woolf's Method** is based on Weighing each stratum according to its sampling error - giving the most weight to those strata that have the smallest variance.

Woolf's Method: In this method, we initially work with log of the odds ratio and the formula uses the weighted average

Data of Woolf's Method will be taken in 2 × 2 contingency

Risk Factor	Disease Status	
	Disease	No Disease
Exposed	a_i	b_i
Not Exposed	c_i	d_i

The steps involved in the computation of Woolf''s method values on the log scale, as explained below

Step 1 - Weighted Average of the Log odds ratio

The log OR of Woolf's method is obtained by the equation $\log\left(\hat{OR}_w\right) = \dfrac{\sum_{i=1}^{I} W_i \log \hat{OR}_i}{\sum_{i=1}^{I} W_i}$,

where W_i s are considered as weight of each stratum and $\log \hat{OR}_i$ the odd ratio of each ith stratum. When the sample size is very small in some stratum, then the investigator use the small sample adjusted estimates, which is given the equation

$$\log\left(\hat{OR}_i\right) = \log\left[\frac{\left(a+\frac{1}{2}\right)\left(d+\frac{1}{2}\right)}{\left(\left(b+\frac{1}{2}\right)\left(c+\frac{1}{2}\right)\right)}\right]$$

The weighted average of the different strata is the weighted average of log odds ratio for each of the strata. In other words, this is the sum of the products of each stratum-specific log odds ratio times its weight, all divided by the sum of the weights.

Pros and Cons of Woolf's Method

Conceptually this method is very straightforward

This method more ideal when the number of strata is small and the sample size within each strata is large

In this method, it is not possible to calculate Woolf's when any one value of a cell in any stratum is zero, because log(0) is undefined

In this method 0.5 cell corrections have been suggested based on the bias

The Wald Method. This is one of the method that will be used to compute a confidence interval for b, this method simply computes the test statistic by dividing the maximum likelihood estimate of b by an estimate of its standard deviation.

In case of null hypothesis, $H_0:b=0$, then the Wald statistic Zb is obtained by the equation $Zb = \dfrac{\hat{b}}{\sqrt{\hat{v}}}$ will approximately follow a standard Normal distribution in large samples. Comparison with tables of the standard Normal distribution thus yields a p-value. Often the Wald statistic is squared and then compared to a λ^2 distribution with one degree of freedom.

Mantel-Haenzel Method

In most of the epidemiological studies, the investigator will be concerned with one outcome variable or event like disease, and a primary risk factor such as an exposure, which causes some harmful effect to the population. We the investigator are aware of another variable, that may be associated with the risk factor, disease or with disease and risk factor. In true sense, the relationship of that variable between risk factor and disease is masked. Such type of factors are called as confounding variable. There are some situations, where the investigator wish to adjust a confounder, which may influence the outcome of a statistical analysis of the experimental data. A confounder is one that may be associated with either disease or exposure or both disease and exposure. Here the investigator will go for different strata of case-control study, then Mantel-Haenszel method will be applied to obtain OR. This methods works well regardless of the sample sizes and Marginal balances in the stratum-Specific 2×2 – tables.

The ODD's at each level of stratum is estimated by $\dfrac{ad}{bc}$, later the Mantel-Haenszel procedure pools the data of different levels of the confounders to compute and that is obtained by the mathematical equation.

$$\mathrm{OR}_{MH} = \frac{\left(\Sigma\left(a_i d_i \,/\, n_1\right)\right)}{\left(\Sigma\left(b_i c_i \,/\, n_i\right)\right)}$$

In order to obtain the confidence interval, we need to use the log scale. In case of Mantel-Haenszel method the $\mathrm{var}(\log(\mathrm{OR}_{MH}))$ is obtained using the mathematical equation

$$\mathrm{var}(\log(\mathrm{OR}_{MH})) =$$

$$\left[\frac{\sum_1^I \left(\dfrac{a_i + d_i}{n_i}\right)\left(\dfrac{a_i d_i}{n_1}\right)}{2\left(\sum_1^I \dfrac{a_i d_i}{n_i}\right)^2} + \frac{\sum_1^I \left(\dfrac{a_i + d_i}{n_i}\cdot\dfrac{b_i c_i}{n_i} + \dfrac{b_i c_i}{n_i}\cdot\dfrac{a_i d_i}{n_i}\right)}{2\left(\sum_1^I \dfrac{a_i d_i}{n_i}\right)\left(\sum_1^I \dfrac{b_i c_i}{n_i}\right)} + \frac{\sum_1^I \left(\dfrac{b_i + c_i}{n_i}\right)\left(\dfrac{b_i c_i}{n_i}\right)}{2\left(\sum_1^I \dfrac{b_i c_i}{n_i}\right)^2} \right]$$

Then the Confidence Interval for 95% level is obtained be the equation

$$\log\left(\mathrm{OR}_{MH}\right) \pm Z\alpha\sqrt{\left(\mathrm{var}\,\log\mathrm{OR}_{MH}\right)}$$

Example: A case control study was conducted to identify the reasons for getting the lung cancer among the residents of coastal city. The primary risk factor under the investigation was found to be due to the employment in a chemical industry and smoking. The data are tabulated separately in three levels as shown in the table

Smoking	Employed in Chemical Industry	Lung cancer	No Lung cancer
No	Yes	11-a	35-b
	No	50-c	203-d
Moderate	Yes	70-a	42-b
	No	217-c	220-d
Heavy	Yes	14-a	3-b
	No	96-c	50-d

Solution:

Smoking	Employed in Chemical Industry	Lung cancer	No Lung cancer	Total
No	Yes	11	35	46
	No	50	203	253
	Total	61	238	299
Moderate	Yes	70	42	112
	No	217	220	437
	Total	287	262	549
Heavy	Yes	14	3	17
	No	96	50	146
		110	53	163

No smoking and Lung Cancer

$a = 11$

$$\frac{r_1 c_1}{n} = \frac{(46)(61)}{299} = 9.38$$

$$\frac{r_1 r_2 c_1 c_2}{n^2 (n-1)} = \frac{46 \times 253 \times 61 \times 238}{299^2 (299-1)} = 6.34$$

$$\frac{ad}{n} = \frac{11 \times 203}{299} = 7.47$$

$$\frac{bc}{n} = \frac{35 \times 50}{299} = 5.85$$

Moderate smoking and Lung Cancer

$$a = 70$$

$$\frac{r_1 c_1}{n} = \frac{(112)(287)}{549} = 58.55$$

$$\frac{r_1 r_2 c_1 c_2}{n^2(n-1)} = \frac{112 \times 437 \times 287 \times 262}{549^2(549-1)} = 22.28$$

$$\frac{ad}{n} = \frac{70 \times 287}{549} = 28.05$$

$$\frac{bc}{n} = \frac{42 \times 217}{549} = 16.60$$

Heavy Smokers and Lung cancer

$$a = 14$$

$$\frac{r_1 c_1}{n} = \frac{(17)(110)}{163} = 14.47$$

$$\frac{r_1 r_2 c_1 c_2}{n^2(n-1)} = \frac{17 \times 146 \times 110 \times 53}{163^2(163-1)} = 3.36$$

$$\frac{ad}{n} = \frac{14 \times 50}{163} = 4.29$$

$$\frac{bc}{n} = \frac{3 \times 96}{163} = 1.77$$

$$Z = \frac{\sum a - \sum \left(\dfrac{r_1 c_1}{n}\right)}{\sqrt{\sum \left(\dfrac{r_1 r_2 c_1 c_2}{n^2(n-1)}\right)}} = \frac{(11-9.38)+(70-58.55)+(14-11.47)}{\sqrt{6.34+22.28+3.36}} = 2.76$$

$$OR_{MH} = \frac{\sum \dfrac{ad}{n}}{\sum \dfrac{bc}{n}} = \frac{7.47+28.05+4.29}{5.85+16.60+1.77} = 1.64$$

Application of Mantel-Haenszel

The subjects chosen for the study are stratified according to the different types of confounder and to verify the level of significance difference between disease status and suspected risk factor status in the population which has been selected for the epidemiological study.

Risk Factor	Disease Status		Total
	Case	Control	
Present	a_i	b_i	a_i+b_i
Absent	c_i	d_i	c_i+d_i
	a_i+c_i	b_i+d_i	$n_i=(a_i+b_i)+(c_i+d_i)$

Steps to Compute λ^2_{MH} :

1. Form different strata of icon founding variables

2. For each stratum obtain predicted frequency of the upper left-hand cell (For the variable a_i, corresponding predicted variable $e_i = ((a_i + b_i)\times(a_i + c_i))/n_i$

3. v_i–variance for each is obtained using the equation $vi = (a_i + b_i)(c_i + d_i)(a_i + c_i)(b_i + d_i)/ n_i^2 \times (n_i - 1))$

4. Then the MH –test statistic λ^2_{MH} is computed using the equation

$$\lambda^2_{MH} = \frac{\left(\sum_{i=1}^{I} a_i - \sum_{i=2}^{I} e_i\right)^2}{\sum_{i=1}^{I} v_i}$$

The null hypothesis is rejected, and alternative hypothesis is accepted, when there is an association between disease and risk factor. This can be verified when the computed value of test statistics is greater than the tabulated value of Chi-square for the degree of freedom 1 for the 5% or 1% level of significance.

Example: Data collected by an investigator on obstructive coronary artery disease (OCAD), hypertension and age among the subjects identified to measure association between the Risk Factor, Confounder and Disease (Outcome-OCAD-Case or No-Case) as listed in the table. The data is stratified into two groups as age ≤ 65 and Age > 65. Compute λ^2_{MH} and OR_{MH}

Stratum -1

Risk Factor Hypertension	AGE ≤ 55		Total
	Case (OCAD)	Control (No OCAD)	
Present	19	13	32
Absent	17	5	22
Total	36	18	54

Stratum -2

Risk Factor Hypertension	AGE > 55		Total
	Case (OCAD)	Control (No OCAD)	
Present	52	13	65
Absent	16	7	23
Total	68	20	88

Solution:

$$e_1 = ((a_1+b_1) \times (a_1+c_1))/ n_1 = (36 \times 32)/54 = 21.33$$

$$v_1 = (a_1+b_1)(c_1+d_1)(a_1+c_1)(b_1+d_1)/ n_1^2 \times (n_1 - 1)) = 2.95$$

$$e_2 = ((a_2+b_2) \times (a_2+c_2))/ n_2 = (36 \times 32)/54 = 50.23$$

$$v_2 = (a_2+b_2)(c_2+d_2)(a_2+c_2)(b_2+d_2)/ n_2^2 \times (n_2 - 1)) = 3.02$$

$$\lambda_{MH}^2 = \frac{\left(\sum_{i=1}^{I} a_i - \sum_{i=2}^{I} e_i\right)^2}{\sum_{i=1}^{I} v_i} = \frac{((19+52)-(21.33+20.23))^2}{54+88} = 0.05$$

$$\text{Degree of freedom} = (r-1)(c-1) = (2-1)(2-1) = 1$$

For degree of freedom 1 the tabulated value at 95% level of confidence λ^2 is equal to 3.841. The calculate is less than the table value. There is no association between Confounder (Age), Risk factor (Hypertension) and Disease (OCAD).

Cochran – Mantel – Haenszel Test

This statistical test is applied or used to analyze the data, when the stratified or Matched categorical data are collected. It helps the investigator to test the association level between the predictor or treatment and outcomes which are in the state of Binary like Case and Control. Here we are going to consider the Exposure variable (E) and Non-exposure variable ($\overline{E}$), and the outcome events D (disease is there), $\overline{D}$ (No Disease), by having different stratification. This method of test can be applied for the categorical response. It is often used in observational study, when the subjects are assigned to different treatments, cannot be controlled, but confounding covariates can be measured.

Generally, the investigator considers the binary outcome variables, such as Case (lung cancer) and Binary Predictor variable such as treatment (Smoking). Here the investigator stratifies the data into different strata. later all the stratified data are summarized into 2x2 – contingency table,

Each strata will have one 2x2 – contingency table as shown below

Disease Groups	Treatment Status		Total
	Treatment	**No Treatment**	
Case	a_i	b_i	$N_{1i} = a_i + b_i$
Control	c_i	d_i	$N_{2i} = c_i + d_i$
	$M_{1i} = a_i + c_i$	$M_{2i} = b_i + d_i$	$T_i = (a_i + b_i) + (c_i + d_i)$

Then the odd – ratios of each strata are obtained using the OR $= \dfrac{ad}{bc}$, then the odd – ratio which is common for all strata can be obtained using the Mantel-Haenszel equation $OR_{MH} =$

$$\frac{\left(\sum (a_i d_i / T_1) \right)}{\left(\sum (b_i c_i / T_i) \right)}$$

Then λ^2_{MH} is obtained by using the mathematical equation $\lambda^2_{CMH} \dfrac{\left(\sum_{i=1}^{I} a_i - \sum_{i=1}^{I} N_{1i} M_{1i} / T_i \right)^2}{\sum_{i=1}^{I} \dfrac{N_{1i} N_{2i} M_{1i} M_{2i}}{T_i^2 (T_i - 1)}}$.

When the investigator sets the Null Hypothesis H_0 – that, there is no association between the treatment and outcome i.e., H_0: R = 1. If the hypothesis is against H_0, then the investigator set alternative hypothesis, $H_1 = R \neq 1$.

Each strata of Cochran – Mantel – Haenszel test follows the Chi-Square distribution, then the computed value of λ^2_{CMH} will be compared with the standard tabulated value of λ^2 at 95% percent of confidence for the degree of freedom 1.

Example: A case-Control study was conducted by an investigator in a groups of 400 men aged 40 years and above to measure the relationship between alcohol consumption and liver cancer. In this case smoking variable has been considered as confounder. Perform statistical analysis to measure the association for the Data collected as per two stratification and verify the level of significance.

Alcohol Drinker (Smoking)	Liver Cancer		
		YES	**NO**
	YES	93	65
	NO	24	18

Alcohol Drinker (Non Smoking)	Liver Cancer		
		YES	**NO**
	YES	45	54
	NO	39	64

Solution:

		LIVER CANCER		
Alcohol Drinker		**YES**	**NO**	**Total**
(Smoking)	YES	93	65	158
	NO	24	18	42
Total		117	83	200

		LIVER CANCER		
Alcohol Drinker		**YES**	**NO**	**Total**
(Non Smoking)	YES	45	54	99
	NO	39	62	101

$$e_1 = ((a_1+b_1) \times (a_1+c_1))/ n_1 = (158 \times 117)/200 = 92.43$$

$$v_1 = (a_1+b_1)(c_1+d_1)(a_1+c_1)(b_1+d_1)/ n_1^2 \times (n_1 -1) = 8.10$$

$$e_2 = ((a_2+b_2) \times (a_2+c_2))/ n_2 = (36 \times 32)/54 = 41.58$$

$$v_2 = (a_2+b_2)(c_2+d_2)(a_2+c_2)(b_2+d_2)/ n_2^2 \times (n_2 -1) = 12.21$$

$$\lambda_{CMH}^2 = \frac{\left(\sum_{i=1}^{I} a_i - \sum_{i=2}^{I} e_i\right)^2}{\sum_{i=1}^{I} v_i} = \frac{\left((93+45)-(92.43+41.58)\right)^2}{8.51+12.21} = 0.7828$$

Degree of freedom $= (r-1)(c-1) = (2-1)(2-1) = 1$

Test value is less than the table at 5% level of significance.

OR(SMOKERS) = 1.073

OR(Non Smokers) = 1.33

Obtain var(log(OR$_{MH}$)) is obtained by using the mathematical equation

$$\text{var}\left(\log\left(OR_{MH}\right)\right) = \frac{\sum_{1}^{I}\left(\frac{a_i+d_1}{n_i}\right)\left(\frac{a_i d_i}{n_1}\right)}{2\left(\sum_{1}^{I}\frac{a_i d_i}{n_i}\right)} + \frac{\sum_{1}^{I}\left(\frac{a_i+d_1}{n_i}\cdot\frac{b_i c_i}{n_i} + \frac{b_i+c_1}{n_i}\cdot\frac{a_i d_i}{n_i}\right)}{2\left(\sum_{1}^{I}\frac{a_i d_i}{n_i}\right)\left(\sum_{1}^{I}\frac{b_i c_i}{n_i}\right)} + \frac{\sum_{1}^{I}\left(\frac{b_i+c_i}{n_i}\right)\left(\frac{b_i c_i}{n_i}\right)}{2\left(\sum_{1}^{I}\frac{b_i c_i}{n_i}\right)^2}$$

$$= 0.049$$

Then the Confidence Interval for 95% level is obtained be the equation

$$OR_{MH} = \frac{\left(\Sigma(a_i d_i / n_1)\right)}{\left(\Sigma(b_i c_i / n_i)\right)} = 1.22$$

$$\log\left(OR_{MH}\right) \pm Z\alpha\sqrt{\left(\text{var}\log\left(OR_{MH}\right)\right)} = \ln\left(1.22\right) \pm 1.96 \times \sqrt{0.049}$$

$$U = 0.63$$

$$L = -0.24$$

After Taking exponential Lower limit L = 0.7881 and Upper limit U = 1.8812

CHAPTER 6

Statistical Hypothesis

A statistical Hypothesis is some assumption or statement, which may or may not be true about a population or equivalently about the probability distribution characterizing the given phenomenon, in which we are interested to test on the basis of some evidence from a random sample chosen from that particular population.

In context of sampling from a normal population $N(\mu, \sigma^2)$, then the hypothesis can be written as;

$$H: \mu = \mu_0 \text{ and } \sigma^2 = \sigma_0^2$$

The test of a statistical Hypothesis is a two-way action of taking decision, after observing the experimental results of a random sample taken from the known population. The two-way action may be the acceptance or rejection of the Hypothesis under consideration.

Example: A physician may make statement hypothesize that a certain drug will be effective in 90 percent of the cases for which it has been tested. That hypothesis is one that determines whether or not such statement is true or not with the available experimental result or data.

Tests of Significance

By using the statistics of the sampling distribution, investigator can find the probability that a sample statistic ($\bar{x}$, s^2 etc) would differ from a given hypothetical value of the parameter or from another sample value, by more than a certain amount and hence to answer the question of significance.

Accordingly, a procedure which has been followed to assess the significance of a statistics or difference between the two or more independent statistics is termed as or known as tests of significance.

To perform these tests of significance, depending on the type of clinical or interventional study or based on the problem in which investigator doing experiments, different statistical tests like t-test, ANOVA, Chi-Square test etc., will be applied to test the significance of the parameter of population with sample statistics.

Types of Hypothesis

After selecting the random sample from a given population with a particular characteristic, makes the tests of significance valid for an investigator, who will be doing experiments on animals or patients.

Before applying any test of significance, investigator must set up a hypothesis, that is a definite statement about the population parameter(s) like mean, standard deviation.

Null Hypothesis (H₀)

Such a statistical hypothesis, which is under test, is usually considered as hypothesis of no difference and it is named as null hypothesis and that is denoted as H_0.

In General, null hypothesis can be defined as "Hypothesis which is tested for possible rejection under the assumption that is true".

OR

Hypothesis to be tested for possible rejection or acceptance is also named as Null Hypothesis.

Alternative Hypothesis

Any hypothesis which is against to the hypothesis or hypothesis which is complementary to the null hypothesis is called as alternative hypothesis. It is very important to explicitly state the alternative hypothesis in respect of any null hypothesis H_0.

Rules for Stating Statistical Hypothesis

When hypothesis are considered in any study, then the indication of equality (either =, $\leq$ or $\geq$) must appear in the null Hypothesis.

Example: Average height for certain population is not 66", then null Hypothesis

$H_0 : \mu = 64$" and the alternative Hypothesis $H_1: \mu \# 64$"

1. Suppose , if we want to conclude that population average is greater than 64" then

   $H_0 : \mu \leq 64$" then $H_1 > 64$"

2. If we conclude that the population mean is less than 64", then hypothesis can be written as

3. $H_0 : \mu \geq 64$" then $H_1 < 64$"

Example:

1. When we say that a patient is free from any disease, that is H_0 is true.

2. After conducting or performing pathological test, doctor gives conclusion that patient is free from the disease, then H_0 is true, then H_0 will be accepted, that there is no difference between population mean and sample mean. i.e., $\mu = \mu_0$.

3. If a patient is having any disease, conclusion will be against to the null hypothesis, then alternative hypothesis is true. H_1 is accepted. Population mean is not equal to H_0, $\mu \# \mu_0$.

Types of Error in Testing Hypothesis

In any experimental study, the inference consists of coming to the conclusion to accept or reject null Hypothesis (H_0) after observing the result obtained from a random sample taken from the population. There are chances of taking wrong decisions about the result obtained or on the Hypothetical statement. There are four possibilities to make decision about the result obtained from the random sample. The decisions are:

  (i)   Reject H_0 when H_0 is true is false

  (ii) Accept H_0 when H_0 is true is true

  (iii) Reject H_0 when H_0 is true is true

  (iv) Accept H_0 when H_0 is true is false

Example:

1.   When patient is not free from disease, H_0 is not true, reject H_0 – decision is correct.

2.   When patient is free from disease, H_0 is true, accept H_0 – decision is correct.

3.   When patient is free from disease, H_0 is true, but the investigator reject H_0 – decision is incorrect.

4.   When patient is not free from disease, H_0 is not true, but the investigator or test result says, he is free from the disease, accepts H_0 – decision is incorrect.

There are two possible errors which will be committed by the investigators, they are named as Type-I and Type-II error.

Type-I – Error: The error of rejecting H_0 when H_0 is true is known as Type-I error.

TYPE-II – Error: The error of accepting H_0 , when H_0 is false or rejecting H_1 , when H_1 is true is known as Type-II.

Those decision can be shown in the table form

Condition of Null Hypothesis

		True	False
Possible Actions	Reject H_1 when H_1 - true	Correct Action	Type – II Error
	Reject H_0 when H_0 - True	Type-I Error	Correct action

Note: Investigator makes Type-I Error by rejecting H_0 and Type-II-Error by rejecting H_1 when H_0 and H_1 are true. These two errors can be written as

$$P \text{ [Reject } H_0 \text{ when } H_0 \text{ is true]} = P[\text{Type} - \text{I Error}] = \alpha$$

$$P \text{ [Reject } H_1 \text{ when } H_1 \text{ is true or Accepting } H_0 \text{ when } H_0 \text{ is not true]}$$

$$= P \text{ [Type} - \text{II} - \text{Error]} = \beta$$

In the terminology of clinical trial

$$\alpha = P \text{ [Rejecting healthy patients]}$$

$$\beta = P \text{ [Rejecting diseased patients]}$$

Power of Test

According to the hypothetical statement β can be written as

$\beta = P\,[\text{Type} - \text{II} - \text{Error}]$

$\quad = P\,[\text{Accepting } H_0 \text{ when } H_0 \text{ is not true}]$

But according to theory of probability, if p is probability of success and q – is probability of failure, then $p + q = 1$

$\therefore$ P [Accepting H_0 when H_0 is not true] + P [Accepting H_0 when H_0 is true] = 1

$\beta + \alpha = 1$

$\alpha = 1 - \beta$

$1 - \beta = P\,[\text{Accepting } H_0 \text{ when } H_0 \text{ is true}]$ is called as the power of tests

Hence, minimizing β, results in maximizing $(1 - \beta)$, which is called as power of test. In the usual practice of the study or testing the hypothesis, the α will be fixed and then try to obtain a criterion to minimize β.

For any given statistical test α is a single number, which will be assigned by an investigator before performing any test or clinical trial experiment. It is also named as acceptable risk of rejecting a true null hypothesis.

On the other hand, β may assume one of many values. If we wish to test the null hypothesis, that some population parameter is equal to some specified value. If H_0 is false and we fail to reject it, then the investigator will commit type-II error. This depends on

(a) The actual or true value of the parameter of interest.
(b) The hypothesized value of the parameter.
(c) The value of α and
(d) The sample size n.

When H_0 is false, the investigator would like to know, what could be the probability that one can reject that. The information can be obtained by using power of test, which is written as $1-\beta$. The value $(1-\beta)$ is the probability, which can reject the false null hypothesis. The $1-\beta$. Can take correct action when H_0 is false. The result can be called as a power of function.

Level of Significance

The maximum size of type-I error, where the investigator prepared to risk is known as the level of significance. The level of significance is denoted as α and commonly used level of significance are 5% (0.05) and 1% (0.01).

OR

The significance level is the probability of rejecting the null hypothesis when it is true. For example, a significance level of 0.05 indicates a 5% risk of concluding that a difference exists when there is no actual difference.

When we say 5% level of significance, it implies that 5 samples out of 100, we are likely to reject. In other way, that the investigators are 95% confident, that the decision taken to reject H_0 is correct. In any statistical calculation or analysis that is always fixed in advance, before collecting the information about the sample which we are going to be selected for experimental study.

Critical Region

When an investigator takes several samples of same from a particular population, on which experimental study has to be performed and compute some statistics t (say $\bar{x}$, p etc) for each sample. The statistics of each samples (t_1, t_2, t_3-----t_k) may be used to test some null hypothesis. Some statistics of these samples may lead to rejection of H_0 and other may lead to acceptance of H_0. The statistics which leads to the rejection of H_0 is called as critical region (C) or rejection region (R), and statistics which leads to the acceptance of H_0 can be called as Acceptance region (A).

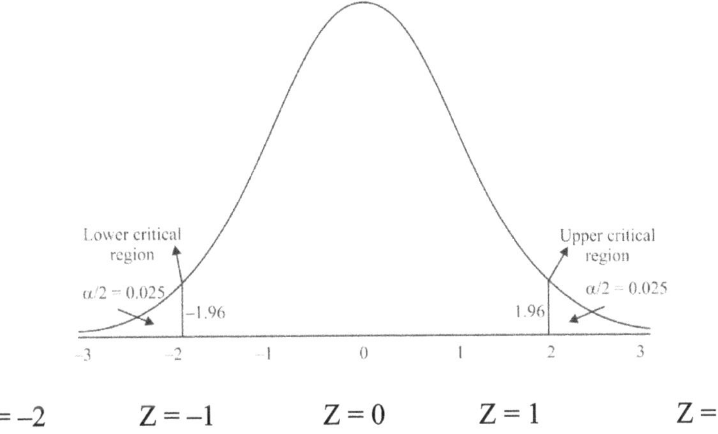

$$Z = -2 \qquad Z = -1 \qquad Z = 0 \qquad Z = 1 \qquad Z = 2$$

The critical region for two tailed test at the level of significance α is given by $Z > Z_{\alpha/2}$ or

$$Z < -Z_{\alpha/2}$$

Right tailed test

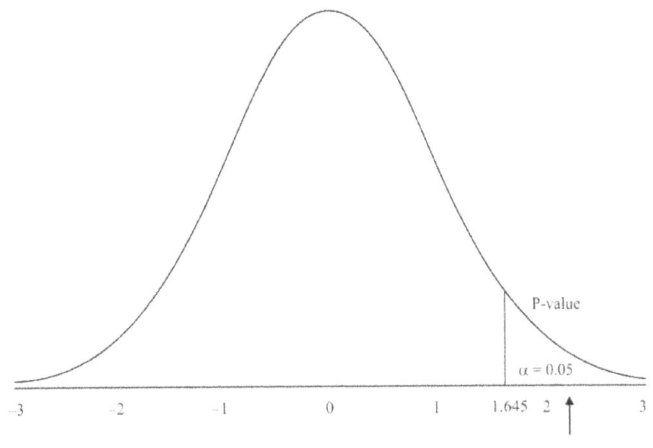

Left tailed test

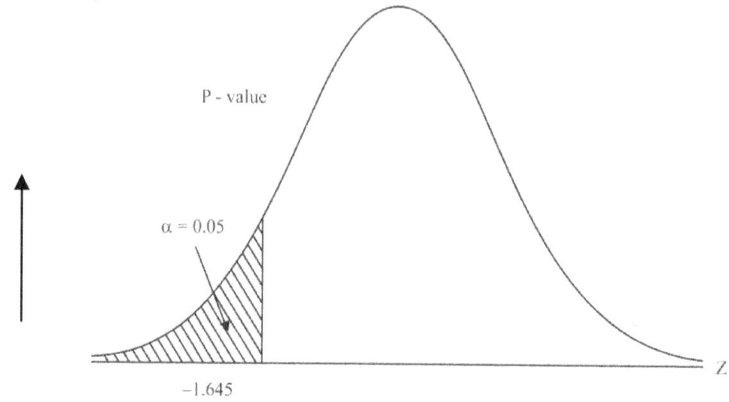

The critical (rejection) region at the level of significance α is

(i) $Z > Z\,\alpha$ for right tailed test

(ii) $Z < -Z\,\alpha$ for left tailed test

P-Values

The level of statistical significance is often expressed as a p-value between 0 and 1. The smaller the p-value, the stronger the evidence that you should reject the null hypothesis. A p-value less than 0.05 (typically ≤ 0.05) is statistically significant.

Instead of making a statement on the experimental or observed value of the test – statistics is significant or not, many investigators writes in their research paper to write report of the result in terms P value. The P-value is the level of marginal significance within a statistical hypothesis test representing the probability of the occurrence of a given event. The p-value is used as an alternative to rejection points to provide the smallest level of significance at which the null hypothesis would be rejected.

Probability of getting values of the test statistics as extreme as or more extreme than, that observed if the null hypothesis is true.

When $P < \alpha$, H_0 is rejected

$P \geq \alpha$, H_0 is not rejected.

However, the reporting of P-values as part of the results of an investigation is more informative to the readers than statements such as "the null Hypothesis is rejected at the level of 0.05 or 5%" or "the results are not significant at the level of 0.05 or 5%".

P-Value testing Method

The level at which the test is significant, then that is given as probability, rather than percentage and that is called as p – value. The p value is the exact probability of getting a result as extreme as that observed for the test statistic when null hypothesis is true.

Step 1: Compute from the observations, the observed value t_{obs} of the test statistic T.

Step 2: Calculate the p-value. This is the probability, under the null hypothesis, of sampling a test statistic at least as extreme as that which was observed.

Step 3: Reject the null hypothesis, in favor of the alternative hypothesis, if and only if the p-value is less than the significance level (the selected probability) threshold.

The two processes are equivalent. The former process was advantageous in the past when only tables of test statistics at common probability thresholds were available. It allowed a decision to be made without the calculation of a probability. It was adequate for class work and for operational use, but it was deficient for reporting results.

The latter process relied on extensive tables or on computational support not always available. The explicit calculation of a probability is useful for reporting. The calculations are now trivially performed with appropriate software.

Testing of Hypothesis

Tests of Significance for a Single Mean

If x_1, x_2,.......x_n are the n-observations of the sample or n-subjects who have been taken for study, these subjects are selected in a random way from the population whose mean is μ and standard deviation is σ

then

$$|Z| = \frac{|\overline{x} - \mu|}{\sigma / \sqrt{n}}$$

$\overline{x}$ is the mean or average of the sample chosen from / drawn from large population.

Note:

1. If the standard deviation of population is not known then $\sigma = s$, s – standard deviation of sample

2. Confidence limits for μ

   For 95 and 99% confidence limits can be obtained for population mean μ using the equations

   For 95% Confidence limits: $\overline{x} \pm 1.96 \ \sigma/n$ or $\overline{x} \pm 1.96 \ s/\sqrt{n}$

   For 99% Confidence limits: $\overline{x} \pm 2.58 \ \sigma/n$ or $\overline{x} \pm 2.58 \ s/\sqrt{n}$

Tests of Significance for Difference of Means

The tests of significance between the means of two large samples can be obtained by the equation

$$Z = \frac{\overline{x1} - \overline{x2}}{\sqrt{\sigma\left(\frac{1}{n_1} + \frac{1}{n_2}\right)}}$$ where $\overline{x1}$ is the mean sample 1 chosen from population 1 and $\overline{x2}$ is the mean

sample$_1$ chosen from population 2. Here both the samples are taken from very large populations.

$$s = \sqrt{\frac{n_1 s_1^{\,2} + n_2 s_2^{\,2}}{n_1 + n_2}}$$

s is combined standard deviation of two samples which are chosen from two large populations. If σ - standard deviation of the population is not known, then $s = \sigma$

Comparision of Two Proportions

In case of categorical data, common problem an investigator can encounter is comparing the two proportions. In this study we will have two independent samples of binary data (n_1, x_1) and (n_2, x_2), n_1 and n_2 are sizes of two samples, they may be equal and x_1 and x_2 are number of positive outcomes of two samples.

To analyze the data, steps involved are.

1. Consider null hypothesis H_0: $P_1 = P_2$ for two tailed test.

2. Chose the level of significance $\alpha = 0.05$ (95% confidence level)

3. Compute $Z = \dfrac{p_1 - p_2}{\sqrt{p(1-p)\left(\dfrac{1}{n_1} + \dfrac{1}{n_2}\right)}}$

Where $P = \dfrac{x_1 + x_2}{n_1 + n_2}$

This is an estimate of common proportion under H_0

For two tailed test H_1: $p_1 \neq p_2$ $Z < 1.96$ or $Z > 1.96$

The term $p_2 - p_1$ measures the difference between two samples. If we assume H_0 then $p_2 - p_1 = 0$

Under H_0

The denominator of Z is the standard error of $p_2 - p_1$, a measure of how good $p_2 - p_1$ is an estimate of $P_2 - P_1$

The Z is a value, that indicates $p_2 - p_1$ is significant or not .

Very Z is denoted by X^2 and it is obtained by the equation,

$$x^2 = \frac{(n_1 + n_2)\left[x_1(n_2 - x_1) - x_2(n_1 - x_1)\right]^2}{n_1 n_2 (x_1 + x_2)(n_1 + n_2 - x_2 - x_1)}$$

The Null hypothesis is rejected at the level of significance $\alpha = 0.05$ $X^2 \geq 3.84$ for DOF $= 1$

When data is 2×2 contingency table then $\lambda^2 = \dfrac{(a+b+c+d)(ad - bc^2)}{(a+c)(b+c)(a+b)(c+d)}$

Example: Clinical trial experiment was performed by an investigator to verify the fatal Poisoning of children using two drugs A and B, which are root cause for deaths. In both case survey was done to verify how a child had received the fatal overdose and responsibility for the accident as assessed. The data collected is as listed below.

	Drug A	Drug B
Child Respond	8	12
No Respond	31	19
	39	31

Solution:

$$P_1 = \frac{8}{8+31} = 0.205$$

$$P_2 = \frac{12}{12+19} = 0.388$$

$$\lambda^2 = \frac{(a+b+c+d)(ad-bc)^2}{(a+c)(b+c)(a+b)(c+d)} = \frac{(39+31)(8\times19-12831)^2}{39\times31\times20\times30}$$

$$= 2.80 < 3.84$$

The difference is not significant

Example: A case control study was conducted among a groups of woman aged 30 years and more to investigate the relationship between the coffee drinking and osteoporosis. Apply Z- test between the two proportions and verify for level of significance.

	Osteoporosis		
Coffee Drinker	Yes	No	Total
Yes	138 = x_1	118 = x_2	256
No	65	76	141
Total	203	194	397

Solution:

Where $\quad P = \dfrac{x_1 + x_2}{n_1 + n_2}$

P1 = x_1/ n_1 = 138/203 = 0.680, P_2 = x_2/n_2 = 118/194 = 0.608

P = (138 + 118)/ (203 + 194) =0.645

Z Compute $\quad Z = \dfrac{p_1 - p_2}{\sqrt{p(1-p)\left(\dfrac{1}{n_1} + \dfrac{1}{n_2}\right)}} = 1.489 < 1.96,$

difference is not significant between coffee drinker and Osteoporosis

Tests of Significance based on t-Distribution

The significance of the test based on the fundamental assumptions in all the sample test are:

(i) The parent population(s) from which the samples (s) is (are) drawn is (are) normally distributed.

(ii) The samples (s) is (are) random and independent of each other.

The T-distribution is a theoretical probability distribution, and the shape of the distribution will be symmetric and bell shaped and the investigator assumes that the mean of the distribution will equal to mean of the population. In all aspect t-distribution will be similar to standard normal curve, but the difference is that area under the normal curve is more than the t-distribution curve. T-distribution will vary more, because standard deviation S – will vary more from sample to sample, in case of small samples, but S-remains constant for large sample. The variability in the sampling distribution of t depends on the sample size n. As the degree of freedom becomes smaller, then we find more variable in its sampling distribution.

To obtain a confidence interval for population mean μ, two conditions should be satisfied. First condition, the random sample must be taken from the population. Second condition is that the population must be approximately normally distributed.

T-Distribution

The t-distribution is obtained by the equation $t = \dfrac{\left|\overline{x} - \mu\right|}{s}\sqrt{n}$.

In this case, standard deviation of the population will be not known, but the standard deviation of the sample will be obtained by equation $s = \sqrt{\dfrac{\Sigma\left(x - \overline{x}\right)^2}{n-1}}$.

Student's 'T'

Definition

If x_1, x_2 ... x_n is a random sample of size n chosen from a normal population with mean μ and standard deviation s, then student's t-statistic is defined as

$$t = \frac{\left|\overline{x} - \mu\right|}{s}\sqrt{n}$$

where $\overline{x}$ is the mean of sample and standard deviation of the sample. $s = \sqrt{\dfrac{\Sigma\left(x - \overline{x}\right)^2}{n-1}}$.

Since size of the random sample taken for study is small and bias will be there in choosing sample, to reduce bias in random selection of sample, size n is reduced by (n–1), that is also called as degree of freedom and that is denoted as $\lambda = (n–1)$.

Critical Value of T

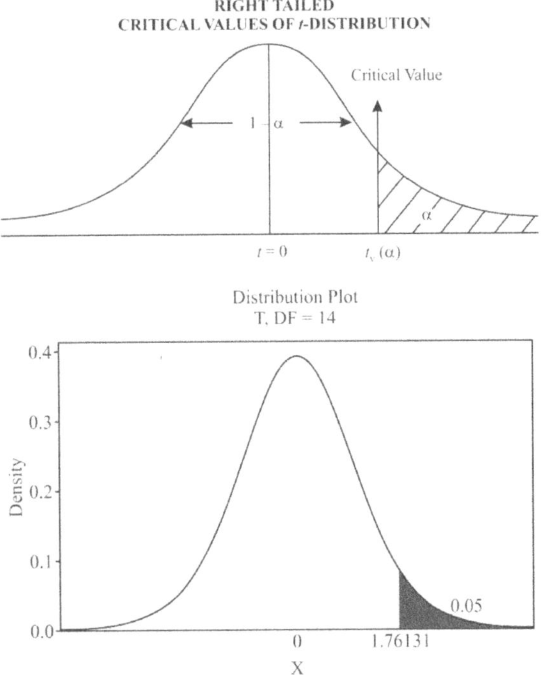

Here we define $P[t > t_\lambda(\alpha)] = \alpha$

The value of $t_\lambda(\alpha)$ is called as the upper (right tailed) – critical (or significant) value of t for (λ = df) and the corresponding confidence coefficient $(1 - \alpha)$

Two Tailed Test

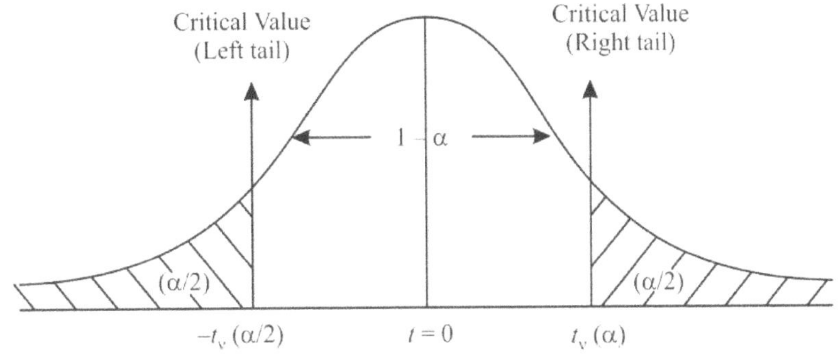

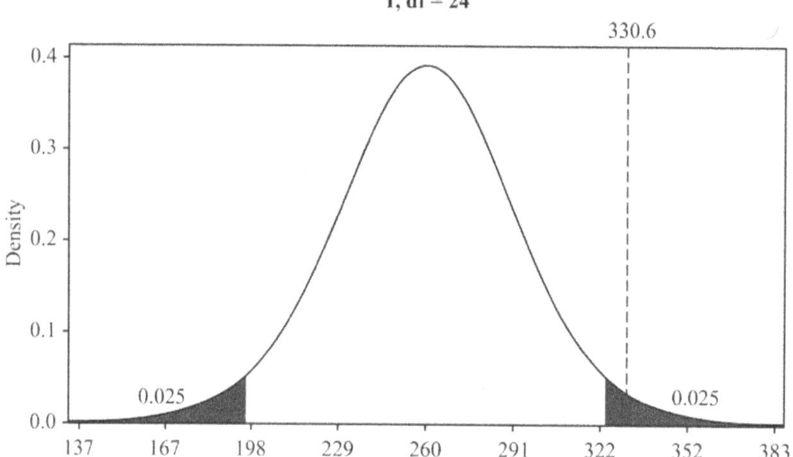

The two tailed critical values of t for degree of freedom λ with equal tails, each of area ($\alpha/2$) are given by $t_\lambda\,(\alpha/2)$: +ve critical value and $-\,t_\lambda\,(\alpha/2)$: -ve critical value. These critical values are tabulated in a t-distribution for different values α and λ.

T-test can be classified into three types, they are:

1. **Sample t-test:** This will be used to know the level of significance between population mean and sample mean or to know that the sample is coming from same population or from different population.

2. **Independent or Unpaired or Pooled sample t-test:** This t-test is most useful to know the level of significant difference between two independent samples which are taken from two different samples.

3. **Comparison or Difference or Paired or Student's t-test:** This test is applied to know the level of significance between the control and treatment, before and after treatment or Treatment and Placebo group.

Inference for a Single Mean

The confidence interval to obtain the range of population mean is $\overline{X}\pm t_{n-1}\dfrac{s}{\sqrt{n}}$, where t_{n-1} is

critical value of 't' at 95% or 99% level of confidence, for the corresponding degree of freedom $(n-1)$. For every sample of size with Degree of Freedom ∞, then 1.96 and 2.58 can be considered as critical values of t at 95% and 99% confidence level.

By applying sample t-test . a hypothesis test for null hypothesis H_0: $\mu = \mu_0$ obtained by the

equation $t = \quad t = \dfrac{|\overline{x}-\mu|}{s}\sqrt{n}$ where $\overline{x}$ is the mean of sample and standard deviation of the

sample. $s = \sqrt{\dfrac{\Sigma\left(x-\overline{x}\right)^2}{n-1}}$.

Comparing Two Mean

When an investigator wish to compare mean values of the same variable between two subgroups of two separate populations, then the two samples should be drawn independently , then they can apply two sampled t-test and the corresponding confidence interval will be obtained using

$$\text{equation } t = \frac{\left|\overline{x_1} - \overline{x_2}\right|}{s}\sqrt{\frac{n_1 \times n_2}{n_1 + n_2}} \text{ where } \overline{x_1} = \frac{\Sigma x_1}{n_1} \text{ and } \overline{x_2} = \frac{\Sigma x_2}{n_2} \text{ and standard deviation}$$

$$s = \sqrt{\frac{\Sigma d_1^2 + \Sigma d_2^2}{n_1 + n_2 - 2}}, \quad \Sigma d_1^2 = \Sigma\left(x_1 - \overline{x}_1\right)^2 \text{ and } \Sigma d_2^2 = \Sigma\left(x_2 - \overline{x}_2\right)^2 \text{ and } (n_1 + n_2 - 2) \text{ is degree of}$$

freedom.

After obtaining the t-value, the computed value will be compared with the table or standard value for the corresponding degree of freedom $\lambda = (n_1 + n_2 - 2)$ at 5% or 1% level of significance to accept or to reject null hypothesis H_0.

Then we can obtain confidence interval for the difference between two population mean

$(\mu_1 - \mu_2)$ is constructed by using the equation $\left[\overline{x1} - \overline{x2} \mp t_{(n1+n2-n)}\left(\alpha/2\right)s\sqrt{\left(\frac{1}{n_1} + \frac{1}{n_2}\right)}\right]$. The $(n_1 +$

$n_2 - 2)$ is degree of freedom, S is combined standard deviation and $t(\alpha/2)$ is the critical value of t for the corresponding degree of freedom at 5% and 1% level of significance.

This procedure is also called as pooled t-test.

The assumption to be made in case of two separate groups are

1. Assume the samples are independent random sample, observation of one group will be not known about the observation of another group.

2. Assume both the populations are normally distributed.

3. Assume standard deviation or variance of both the population or both the groups are equal.

Example: In a group of 40 patient 18 patients of K-L2 staging   and 22 patients of K-L3 stating were treated with Ozone to reduce pain and reduction in pain rate as per the Kellgren-Lawrence scaling is as listed below. Do you find any significance difference between K-L2 and K-L3 stage.?

OZONE					
KL2 - Stage-X1	KL3- Staging-X2	d_1	d_2	d_1^2	d_2^2
3	3	0.28	0.09	0.08	0.01
4	3	1.28	0.09	1.64	0.01
3	4	0.28	1.09	0.08	1.19
2	3	−0.72	0.09	0.52	0.01
3	3	0.28	0.09	0.08	0.01
2	2	−0.72	−0.91	0.52	0.83

Contd...

2	3	−0.72	0.09	0.52	0.01
2	2	−0.72	−0.91	0.52	0.83
3	4	0.28	1.09	0.08	1.19
3	4	0.28	1.09	0.08	1.19
3	3	0.28	0.09	0.08	0.01
2	2	−0.72	−0.91	0.52	0.83
3	3	0.28	0.09	0.08	0.01
3	3	0.28	0.09	0.08	0.01
3	3	0.28	0.09	0.08	0.01
3	2	0.28	−0.91	0.08	0.83
3	2	0.28	−0.91	0.08	0.83
2	3	−0.72	0.09	0.52	0.01
	3		0.09		0.01
	4		1.09		1.19
	3		0.09		0.01
	2		−0.91		0.83
$\sum X1 = 49$	$\sum X12 = 64$			5.61	9.82
N1 = 18	N2 = 22				
$\overline{X1} = \sum X1/N1 = 2.72$	$\overline{X2} = \sum X2/N2 = 2.91$				

$$s = \sqrt{\frac{\Sigma d_1^2 + \Sigma d_2^2}{n_1 + n_2 - 2}}$$

$$t = \frac{\left|\overline{x}_1 - \overline{x}_2\right|}{s} \sqrt{\frac{n_1 \times n_2}{n_1 + n_2}} = 0.923$$

$$DOF = \lambda = N1 + N2 - 2 = 18 + 22 - 2 = 38$$

$$P = 0.361973459 > 0.05$$

Difference is not significant.

Drug has same effect on KL2 and KL3 staging

Paired T-test for the Difference of Means

This paired t-test is also named as comparison, difference and student's t-test. In general this test will be applied to know the level of significance difference between before and after treatment.

Suppose an investigator wants to find whether the drug is really effective in curing the disease or not. Let $x_1, x_2, \ldots x_n$ be the disease status of patients before treatment and $y_1, y_2, \ldots y_n$ be the condition of the disease or disease status of the patients after treatment. In order to test level of significance difference between before and after treatment, we apply paired t-test.

Let $d_i = x_i - y_i$ $(i = 1, 2, \ldots n)$ denote the difference in the observations of subjects or items. The test – value can be computed using the equation

$$t = \frac{\overline{d}}{s}\sqrt{n} \quad \text{where } d = x - y \text{ and } \overline{d} = \frac{\Sigma d}{n} \text{ and } s = \sqrt{\frac{\Sigma d^2 - (\overline{d})^2 \times n}{n-1}}$$

In such cases, the degree of freedom $\lambda = (n - 1)$

Interventional Study

Interventional studies are often prospective and are specifically tailored to evaluate direct impacts of treatment or preventive measures on disease. Each study design has specific outcome measures that rely on the type and quality of data utilized.

This study is also called as clinical trial, and is experiment done on patients, to assess the safety, efficacy and / or the mechanism of action of an investigational medicinal product or procedure, or new drug or device that is in the process of development, but potentially not yet approved by a health authority (e.g. Food and Drug Administration).

To test efficacy of new drug formulation in the treatment of a specific disease, one group of patients are treated new drug and another group will be treated with placebo or standard drug. In this situation both the groups should match each with respect the baseline variable which are measured before assigning them into case group and control group.

The main feature of this interventional study is that the allocation of subjects to treatment is planned and that will be decided and chosen according to randomization.

To analyze the data of interventional study, the paired t-test can be applied, when we go for continuous data and sample size is very small.

Example: In a group of 18 patients of K-L2 staging were treated with Ozone to reduce pain and reduction in pain rate as per the Kellgren-Lawrence scaling is as listed below. Do you find any significance difference between before and after treatment patients in K-L2. stage.?

PRE VAS - Before treatment	6th month VAS - After Treatment
9	2
8	4
8	3
8	3
8	2
8	2
7	2
8	3
9	3
8	3
9	3

Contd...

10	3
5	3
8	3
7	2
9	3
10	3
8	2

Solution:

PRE VAS - Before treatment- B	6th month VAS - After Treatment - A	d = A − B	d^2
9			
8	4	−4	16
8	3	−5	25
8	3	−5	25
8	2	−6	36
8	2	−6	36
7	2	−5	25
8	3	−5	25
9	3	−6	36
8	3	−5	25
9	3	−6	36
10	3	−7	49
5	3	−2	4
8	3	−5	25
7	2	−5	25
9	3	−6	36
10	3	−7	49
8	2	−6	36
		∑d = −98	558

n = Number of subjects =18

Mean = $\overline{d}$ = Σd / N = −98/18 = −5.44

$$SD = s = \sqrt{\frac{\Sigma d^2 - \left(\overline{d}\right)^2 \times n}{n-1}} = \sqrt{\frac{\Sigma 558 - \left(-5.44\right)\hat{2} \times 18}{18-1}} = 1.20$$

$$t = \frac{\overline{d}}{s}\sqrt{n} = \text{abs}\,(-5.44/1.20) \times \sqrt{18} = 19.26$$

$$DOF = \lambda = n - 1 = 18 - 1 = 17$$
$$P = 5.5228E - 13 < 0.05$$

Therefore, the difference is significant between before and after treatment in this interventional study.

Data is analyzed using SPSS statistical software

Paired Samples Statistics		Mean	N	Std. Deviation	Std. Error Mean
Pair 1	BEFORE	8.1667	18	1.15045	.27116
	AFTER	2.7222	18	.57451	.13541

Paired Samples Test									
		Paired Differences					t	df	Sig. (2-tailed)
		Mean	Std. Deviation	Std. Error Mean	95% Confidence Interval of the Difference				
					Lower	Upper			
Pair 1	BEFORE - AFTER	5.44	1.199	.28264	4.84813	6.04076	19.26	17	.000<0.05

Statistical Models

In general statistical model is a mathematical equation which is going to represent the relation between dependent variable or outcome or response variable denoted as Y and one or more independent variables or explanatory variables which are denoted as X.

The Analysis of variance is a powerful statistical tool or one of the models to test the level of significance. Analysis of variance is a general method of analyzing data from designed experiments, whose objective is to compare more than two groups means.

ANOVA is a parametric procedure with some assumption like samples chosen are independent, distribution is normal, and variances are equal. In this section we are discussing important application of ANOVA in epidemiological study.

Assumption for ANOVA Test

ANOVA test is based on the test statistics F (Variance ratio). To verify the validity of F-test. In ANOVA, there are three important assumptions, which we have to consider are:

(i)   The observations made are independent.
(ii) Parent populations are normal, from which the observation or subjects or items are drawn randomly.
(iii) The different treatments chosen, and environmental effects are additive in nature.

Classification of ANOVA

ANOVA is classified into two methods, they are named as:

1. ONE WAY ANOVA

2. TWO WAY ANOVA

1. **ONE WAY ANOVA:** ANOVA also assumes that there will be an equal variance in each of k groups. In general the one way ANOVA is an extension to three or more samples of t-test procedure which is applied for t-test.

In these subjects are assigned randomly and this design called as completely randomized experimental design.

To analyze data the null hypothesis is written as H_0: $\mu_1 = \mu_2 = \mu_3 \ldots \ldots = \mu_k$, where $\mu_1 =$ the mean of treatmant1, $\mu_2 =$ The mean the treatment 2 and so on.

Suppose there are 15 – tablets are available for the comparison of three assay methods, 5-tablets are assigned for each assay. Here one way ANOVA design would result from a random assignment of the tablets into three groups.

The investigator can carry out the test for the equality of several Population (k) means by the rejection region method. The various steps involved in testing hypothesis are as listed below.

Step 1: Compute $G = \Sigma_i \Sigma_j x_{ij}$ = Grand total of the distribution

Step 2: Compute correction factor (CF) = $\dfrac{G^2}{N}$ where $N = n_1 + n_2 + \ldots + n_K$

N = total number of items chosen for study.

Step 3: Computation of raw Sum squares (RSS)

$RSS = \Sigma_i \Sigma_j x^2_{ij}$ = Sum of the squares of all the observations or experimental results

Step 4: Total sum squares = SST = RSS – CF

Step 5: Computation of $T_i = \sum_{j=1}^{nj} x_{ij}$

$T_i =$ The sum of all the observations in the ith class, i=1, 2, 3 ... k

Step 6: Computations of sum of squares between treatments (Columns)

$$SCC = \frac{T1^1}{n_1} + \frac{T2^2}{n_2} + \ldots + \frac{Tk^2}{n_k} - CF$$

Step 7: Sum of the squares due to error. This is denoted as SSE

$$SSE = SST - SSC$$

$$= \text{Total sum squares} - \text{Sum of squares between the treatments.}$$

Step 8: Mean squares between treatment is MSC = $\dfrac{SSC}{k-1}$

K= Number of samples.

Step 9: Mean squares due to error. It is denoted as MSE

$$MSE = \frac{SSE}{N-k}$$

Step 10: Computation of test statistics under H_0:

$$F = \frac{\text{Mean squares between samples or columns}}{\text{Mean squares due to error}}$$

$$F = \frac{MCS}{MSE}$$

Step 11: The computation of degrees of freedom of numerator and denominator value of F -Distribution.

$\lambda_1 = k - 1 = $ DOF of numerator

$\lambda_2 = N - k = $ DOF of denominator

If the computed value of F for the corresponding DOF λ_1 and λ_2 is greater than the table value or critical value of F at a particular level of significance (5% or 1%), then H_0 is rejected at that level of significance, otherwise it may regarded as true.

Step 12: Critical difference between the samples

After the computation of frequency distribution value, result shows the difference is significant between the samples or treatments, then investigator has to verify which sample is more significant among the samples, which are selected randomly for studies.

To perform this, Least Significance difference (LSD) has to be obtained and that has to be compared with the absolute difference between the means of samples. LSD is computed using the equation

LSD = [The critical value of t at the level of significance for DOF (N – K) of mean square due to error] $\times$ S.E$(x_i - x_j)$

$$LSD = t_{(\alpha/2)(N-k)} \sqrt{MSE\left(\frac{1}{n_1} + \frac{1}{n_2}\right)}$$

$t(\alpha/2)$ – t-value for the corresponding degree of freedom N-k, taken from t-distribution table

MSE - Mean sum square due to error

OR

$$LSD = t_{(\alpha/2)(N-k)} \sqrt{MSE\left(\frac{2}{n_i}\right)}, \text{ if } n_i = n_j$$

If the difference $\left|x_i - x_j\right|$ between the means of any two treatments is greater than LSD, it is said to be significant, otherwise it is not significant.

Construction of ANOVA Table for K groups, when the subjects are randomly assigned into different groups of treatment

	Sum of Squares	df	Mean Square	F	Sig.
Between Groups	SSC	K -1	MSC= SSC/K-1	F=MSC/MSE	P-Value
Within Groups (Due to Error)	SSE	N-K	MSE= SSE/N-K		
Total	SST = SSC- SSE	N-1			

The Mathematical model of one way ANOVA can be written as $Y_{ij} = \mu + \tau_j + \in ij$

Observation = overall mean + difference between specific and overall mean + difference between observation and specific mean

$i = 1,2,3,......n_j$ and $j = 1,2,3.....k$

The terms of the model are

1. μ = Denotes Mean of all the k population means and that is named as grand mean

2. τ_j = Denotes the difference between the mean of jth population and grand mean and it is named or termed as treatment effect.

3. $\in_{ij}$ = The amount of difference to which the individual measurement differ from mean of the population and it is called as error term.

***Example* 1:** Data recorded in the following table shows the effect of three types of diet, with reference to the total serum cholesterol (mmol/l) in 21 different subjects and these 21 subjects were randomly assigned into three groups with 7 patients in each group. Verify the level of significance between these three groups using one way ANOVA, which group is more significant and why?

Subject Number	Diet Types		
	Diet 1	Diet 2	Diet 3
1	6.25	5.90	6.10
2	6.43	6.20	5.45
3	6.20	5.82	5.60
4	6.37	6.00	5.80
5	6.10	5.75	5.75
6	6.45	6.12	5.65
7	6.50	6.80	5.63

Solution:

Subject Number	Diet Types		
	Diet 1-X1	Diet 2-X2	Diet 3-X3
1	6.25	5.90	6.10
2	6.43	6.20	5.45
3	6.20	5.82	5.60
4	6.37	6.00	5.80
5	6.10	5.75	5.75
6	6.45	6.12	5.65
7	6.50	6.80	5.63
Total	44.3	42.59	39.98
Mean	6.33	6.08	5.71

X1	$X1^2$	X2	$X2^2$	X3	$X3^2$
6.25	39.0625	5.9	34.81	6.1	37.21
6.43	41.3449	6.2	38.44	5.45	29.7025
6.2	38.44	5.82	33.8724	5.6	31.36
6.37	40.5769	6	36	5.8	33.64
6.1	37.21	5.75	33.0625	5.75	33.0625
6.45	41.6025	6.12	37.4544	5.65	31.9225
6.5	42.25	6.8	46.24	5.63	31.6969
$\sum X1 = 44.3$	$\sum X1^2\ 280.4868$	$\sum X2 = 42.59$	$\sum X2^2\ 259.8793$	$\sum X3 = 39.98$	$\sum X3^2\ 228.5944$
6.33		6.08		5.71	

1. Grand Total = G = $\sum X1 + \sum X2 + \sum X3 = 126.87$
2. Correction Factor = CF = $G^2/N = 16096/21 = 766.48$
3. Raw sum squares = RSS = $\sum X1^2 + \sum X2^2 + \sum X3^2 = 280.4868 + 259.8793 + 228.5944 = 768.96$
4. Total sum Squares = SST = RSS − CF = 768.96 − 766.48 = 2.48
5. Sum of squares between columns or samples = SSC

$$SSC = \left(\left(\frac{\Sigma(X1)^2}{n1}\right) + \left(\frac{\Sigma(X2)^2}{n2}\right) + \left(\frac{\Sigma(X3)^2}{n3}\right)\right) - CF$$

$$= \left(\left(\frac{\Sigma(44.3)^2}{n1}\right) + \left(\frac{\Sigma(42.59)^2}{7}\right) + \left(\frac{\Sigma(39.98)^2}{7}\right)\right) - 766.48 = 1.35$$

6. Sum of squares due to error = SSE

    SSE = SST − SSC = 2.48 − 1.35 = 1.13

7. Mean Squares between columns or treatment = $MSC = \dfrac{SSC}{K-1}$

    K = number of samples taken for study = 3

    $MSC = \dfrac{1.35}{3-1} = 0.676$

8. Mean square due to error = $MSE = \dfrac{SSE}{N-K} = \dfrac{1.13}{21-3}$

    MSE = 0.063

9. Computation of Test value , F − distribution

    F = MSC/MSE = 0.676/0.063 = 10.75

10. Computation of degree of freedom of numerator (MSC) and denominator (MSE) of F-distribution

    $\lambda 1 = K - 1 = 3 - 1 = 2$

    $\lambda 2 = N - k = 21 - 3 = 18$

11. Computed value of F-distribution should be compared with standard table value of F-distribution at 5% or 1% level of significance.

    Here the table value the degree of freedom 2 and 18 is Fble = 3.08

    F = 10.75 >Fble = 3.08,

    Hence the difference is significant between the means of different samples. Null hypothesis is true.

12. When the difference is significant, we need to compute LSD to verify which sample is more

    significant. $LSD = t_{(\alpha/2)(N-k)} \sqrt{MSE\left(\dfrac{2}{n_i}\right)}$, if $n_i = n_j$

    $LSD = 2.10 \times \sqrt{0.063\left(\dfrac{2}{5}\right)} = 0.28$

13. Compare the means of three groups

Mean	Absolute difference between means of any samples	Comparison with LSD	Remark
Mean1 = $\overline{X1}$ = 44.3	$Abs\left(\overline{X1}-\overline{X2}\right)$ = 44.3 − 42.59 = 1.71 $Abs\left(\overline{X1}-\overline{X3}\right)$ = 44.30 - 39.98 = 4.32	1.71> 0.28 = LSD 4.32>0.28 = LSD	Difference is significant
Mean2 = $\overline{X2}$ = 42.59	$Abs\left(\overline{X2}-\overline{X3}\right)$ = 42.59 − 39.98 = 2.61	2.61> 0.28 = LSD	Difference is significant
Mean3 = $\overline{X3}$ = 39.98			

The average value of X3 is less than the remaining two samples, hence X3 is more significant than remaining two samples

***Example* 2:** A study is designed to test whether there is any difference in mean daily calcium intake in adults with normal bone density, adults with osteopenia (a low bone density which may lead to osteoporosis) and adults with osteoporosis.

Adults of 60 years age with normal bone density, osteopenia and osteoporosis are selected at random from hospital records and invited to participate in the study.

Each participant's daily calcium intake is measured based on basis of food intake and supplements. The data recorded is listed below .

Normal Bone Density-X1	Osteopenia –X2	Osteoporosis-X3
1200	1000	890
1000	1100	650
980	700	1100
900	800	900
750	500	400
800	700	350

Is there any significant difference between the mean calcium intake of patients with normal bone density as compared to patients with osteopenia and osteoporosis?

X1	X2	X3	$X1^2$	$X2^2$	$X3^2$
1200	1000	590	1440000	1000000	792100
1000	1100	650	1000000	1210000	422500
980	700	1100	960400	490000	1210000
900	800	900	810000	640000	810000
750	500	400	562500	250000	160000
800	700	350	640000	490000	122500
$\sum X1 = 5630$	$\sum X2 = 4800$	$\sum X3 = 4290$	$\sum X1^2 = 5412900$	$\sum X2^2 = 4080000$	$\sum X3^2 = 3517100$

$N1 = 6$ $N2 = 6$ $N3 = 6$

$G = 14720$

$N = 18$

$RSS = 13010000$, $CF = 12037688.89$

$SST = 972311.1111$, $SSC = 152477.7778$

$SSE = 819833.3333$, $K = 3$

$MSC = SSC/K - 1 = 76238.89$

$MSE = SSE/(N - K) = 54655.55556$

DOF of numerator $\lambda_{nr} = k - 1 = 3 - 1 = 2$

DOF of denominator $\lambda_{dr} = N - k - 18 - 3 = 15$

$F = MSC/MSE = 76238.89/54655.56$

F = 1.395

Fble = The standard value of F = 3.68

F = 1.395 < 3.68 and P = 0.278 > 0.05

Hence the difference is not significant

***Example* 3:** The comparative study of OZONE, PLATELET RICH PLASMA and 25% DEXTROSE in the treatment of Osteoarthritis of the knee joint of KL-2 staging. The comparative study was done with VAS(VISVAS ANLOGUE SCALE) to verify the reduction rate pain. The reduction rate in pain after three month is as listed below. Verify the level of significance between these three drugs using One-Way ANOVA

OZONE	PRA	25% Dextrose
3	3	5
4	2	4
4	2	4
4	2	3
4	4	4
3	4	3
4	3	4
2	4	5
2	3	5
4	4	4
2	4	3
2	4	3
2	5	5
4	2	5
3	5	4
4	4	6
4	2	5
4	3	5

Solution:

X1	X2	X3	$X1^2$	$X2^2$	$X3^2$
3	3	5	9	9	25
4	2	4	16	4	16
4	2	4	16	4	16
4	2	3	16	4	9
4	4	4	16	16	16
3	4	3	9	16	9
4	3	4	16	9	16
2	4	5	4	16	25

Contd…

2	3	5	4	9	25
4	4	4	16	16	16
2	4	3	4	16	9
2	4	3	4	16	9
2	5	5	4	25	25
4	2	5	16	4	25
3	5	4	9	25	16
4	4	6	16	16	36
4	2	5	16	4	25
4	3	5	16	9	25
$\sum X1 = 59$	$\sum X2 = 60$	$\sum X3 = 77$	$\sum X1^2 = 207$	$\sum X2^2 = 218$	$\sum X3^2 = 343$

$n_1 = 18$, $n_2 = 18$, $n_3 = 18$

$G = 196$, $N = 54$, $RSS = 768$

$CF = 711.41$, $SST = 56.59$, $SSC = 11.37$, $SSE = 45.22$

$K = 3$

$MSC = SSC/K - 1 = 5.69$

$MSE = SSE/(N-K) = 0.88671024$

DOF of $\lambda_{NR} = k-1 = 3-1 = 2$

DOF of $\lambda_{DR} = N-k = 54-3 = 51$

$F = MSC/MSE = 6.412$

Fble $= 3.24$

$P = 0.003 < 0.05$

***Example* 4:** The comparative study of OZONE , PLATELET RICH PLASMA and 25% DEXTROSE in the treatment of Osteoarthritis of the knee joint of KL-2 staging . The comparative study was done with WOMAC Score (Western Ontario and McMaster) to verify functionality. The score given for the functionality after three month is as listed below. Verify the level of significance between these three drugs using One-Way ANOVA

OZONE-X1	PRA-X2	25% Dextrose-X3
32	34	38
35	43	40
36	32	36
35	40	36
35	36	36
35	34	36
33	39	36
36	40	36
34	36	36

Contd...

34	32	36
33	34	30
34	36	35
34	36	37
33	32	37
33	36	43
36	30	41
36	42	39
34	34	39

Solution:

X1	X2	X3	$X1^2$	$X2^2$	$X3^2$
32	34	38	1024	1156	1444
35	43	40	1225	1849	1600
36	32	36	1296	1024	1296
35	40	36	1225	1600	1296
35	36	36	1225	1296	1296
35	34	36	1225	1156	1296
33	39	36	1089	1521	1296
36	40	36	1296	1600	1296
34	36	36	1156	1296	1296
34	32	36	1156	1024	1296
33	34	30	1089	1156	900
34	36	35	1156	1296	1225
34	36	37	1156	1296	1369
33	32	37	1089	1024	1369
33	36	43	1089	1296	1849
36	30	41	1296	900	1681
36	42	39	1296	1764	1521
34	34	39	1156	1156	1521
$\sum X1 = 618$	$\sum X2 = 646$	$\sum X3 = 667$	$\sum X1^2 = 21244$	$\sum X2^2 = 23410$	$\sum X2^2 = 24847$

$K = 3$

$n_1 = 18 \quad n_2 = 18 \quad n_3 = 18$

G = Grand total $= 1931$

$N = 54$, RSS $= 69501$, CF $= 69051.13$

SST $= 449.87$, SSC $= 67.15$, SSE $= 382.72$

MSC $= 33.57$, MSE $= 7.50$

$F = 4.47$

The given data is analyzed using SPSS statistical software and result

Descriptive								
Drugs								
	N	**Mean**	**Std. Deviation**	**Std. Error**	**95% Confidence Interval for Mean**		**Minimum**	**Maximum**
					Lower Bound	**Upper Bound**		
1.00	18	34.3333	1.23669	.29149	33.7183	34.9483	32.00	36.00
2.00	18	35.8889	3.64432	.85897	34.0766	37.7012	30.00	43.00
3.00	18	37.0556	2.77536	.65416	35.6754	38.4357	30.00	43.00
Total	54	35.7593	2.91344	.39647	34.9640	36.5545	30.00	43.00

ANOVA					
Drugs					
	Sum of Squares	**df**	**Mean Square**	**F**	**Sig.**
Between Groups	SSC = 67.148	2	33.574	4.474	P =.016<0.05
Within Groups	SSE = 382.722	51	7.504		
Total	449.870	53			

Post Hoc Tests

Multiple Comparisons						
Dependent Variable: Drugs						
LSD						
(I) Group	**(J) Group**	**Mean Difference (I-J)**	**Std. Error**	**Sig.**	**95% Confidence Interval**	
					Lower Bound	**Upper Bound**
1.00	2.00	-1.55556	.91314	.095	-3.3888	.2776
	3.00	-2.72222[*]	.91314	.004	-4.5554	-.8890
2.00	1.00	1.55556	.91314	.095	-.2776	3.3888
	3.00	-1.16667	.91314	.207	-2.9999	.6665
3.00	1.00	2.72222[*]	.91314	.004	.8890	4.5554
	2.00	1.16667	.91314	.207	-.6665	2.9999

The mean difference between these three drugs is significant at the 0.05 level.

The sample 25% Dextrose is more significant and patients functionality is more in third sample.

***Example* 5:** A survey was done by an investigator to verify the level of association between smoking habit and reduce in serum testosterone level (Normal range is 300 to 100 ng/dL) in between the age of 30 to 40. The survey was done on four groups, they are classified as never smoker, Earlier or former smokers, light smokers and chain or heavy smokers. Each group consists of 10 subjects. Apply one — way ANOVA and verify the level of significance between these four groups.

Never Smoker X1	Earlier or Former Smokers X2	Light Smokers X3	Heavy Smokers X4	$X1^2$	$X2^2$	$X3^2$	$x4^2$
400	460	370	440	160000	211600	136900	193600
450	500	420	250	202500	250000	176400	62500
600	510	430	400	360000	260100	184900	160000
560	580	480	270	313600	336400	230400	72900
850	850	760	340	722500	722500	577600	115600
680	720	600	620	462400	518400	360000	384400
960	930	820	470	921600	864900	672400	220900
720	860	720	700	518400	739600	518400	490000
920	760	600	600	846400	577600	360000	360000
870	650	510	540	756900	422500	260100	291600
$\sum X1 = 7010$	$\sum X2 = 6820$	$\sum X3 = 5710$	$\sum X4 = 4630$	$\sum X1^2 =$ 5264300	$\sum X2^2 =$ 4903600	$\sum X3^2 =$ 3477100	$\sum X3^2$ =2351500
$\overline{X1} = 701$	$\overline{X2} = 682$	$\overline{X3} = 571$	$\overline{X4} = 463$				

K= Number of groups = 4

$n_1 = 10$, $n_2 = 10$, $n_3 = 10$, $n_4 = 10$

Applying the methodology of One-Way ANOVA the following values computed and verified the level of significance

G = Grand total= 24170

N = Total number of Patients =40

RSS = Raw sum squares = 15996500.00

CF= Correction Factor = 14604722.50

SST = Total sum squares = 1391777.50

SSC = Sum of squares between samples = 364627.50

SSE = Sum of squares within samples = 1027150.00

MSC = Mean squares between samples = 121542.50

MSE = Mean squares within samples = 28531.95

F = MSC/MSE= F =4.26

P = 0.011 < 0.05

Data is analyzed using SPSS-22 statistical software

					95% Confidence Interval for Mean				
Group	**N**	**Mean**	**Standard Deviation**	**Standard. Error**	**Lower Bound**	**Upper Bound**	**Minimum**	**Maximum**
1.	10	701.00	197.28	62.38	559.87	842.12	400.00	960.00
2.	10	682.00	167.45	52.95	562.21	801.78	460.00	930.00
3.	10	571.00	155.16	49.06	460. 05	681.99	370.00	820.00
4.	10	463.00	151.95	48.05	354.29	571.70	250.00	700.00
Total	40	604.25	188.90	29.86	543.83	664.66	250.00	960.00

ANOVA

	Sum of Squares	df	Mean Square	F	Sig.
Between Groups	364627.500	3	121542.500	4.260	.011
Within Groups	1027150.000	36	28531.944		
Total	1391777.500	39			

Chi-Square Distribution

The square of a standard normal variable is called as a Chi-square variate with 1 degree of freedom (DOF). If X is a random variable following normal distribution with mean μ and standard deviation σ, then $\left(\dfrac{X-\mu}{\sigma}\right)$ is a standard normal variate $\left(\dfrac{X-\mu}{\sigma}\right)^2$ is called as Chi-Square variate with DOF 1.

If we take $x_1, x_2, x_3, \ldots\ldots\ldots\ldots x_n$ are n-independent variables, having normal distribution with average (Mean) μ_1, μ_2, μ_3 ------- μ_n and standard deviations $\sigma_1, \sigma_2, \sigma_3,$ ------- σ_n are standard deviations. Then the variate $\lambda^2 = \left(\dfrac{X_1-\mu_1}{\sigma_1}\right) + \left(\dfrac{X_2-\mu_2}{\sigma_2}\right) \ldots + \left(\dfrac{X_n-\mu_n}{\sigma_n}\right)^2 = \sum_{i=1}^{n}\left(\dfrac{X_i-\mu_i}{\sigma_i}\right)^2$ which is the sum of the squares of n-independent standard normal variates, this follows Chi-square distribution with n-DOF.

Chi-Square test: This is one the most useful test which was introduced in the year 1900 by Karl Pearson. This is one of the simplest and most widely used non-parametric test in standard analysis. Chi-Square test is used for measuring the significance of the difference between an observed statistical distribution and theoretical distribution. This test is also known as λ^2 _ test of goodness of fit. This will be used to test, if the deviation between observation (experiment) and theory may be attributed to chance (fluctuations of sampling).

Under null hypothesis, that there is no significant difference between the observed (experimental) and the theoretical or hypothetical value, i.e., there is good compatibility between theory and experiment, Karl Pearson proved that the statistic $\lambda^2 = \sum_{i=1}^{n}\left(\dfrac{O_i-Ei}{Ei}\right)^2 = \dfrac{(O_1-E1)^2}{E1} +$

$\dfrac{(O_2 - E2)^2}{E2} + .. + \dfrac{(O_n - En)^2}{En}$ follows λ^2 distribution with $v = n - 1$ DOF, where $O_1, O_2 ... O_n$ are the observed frequencies and E1, E2, ... En are corresponding expected or theoretical frequencies obtained under some theory or hypothesis.

Steps for computation of λ^2 and drawing conclusions:

(i) Compute the expected frequencies E1, E2, ..., En corresponding to the corresponding observed frequencies $O_1, O_2, ... O_n$ under some theory or hypothesis.

(ii) Compute the deviations (O-E) for each frequency and then square them to obtain $(O - E)^2$.

(iii) Divide the square of the deviations $(O - E)^2$ by the corresponding expected frequency to find $(O-E)^2/E$.

(iv) Obtain $\lambda^2 = \Sigma \left[\dfrac{(O - E)^2}{E} \right]$

(v) Assume Null Hypothesis (H_0). The theory fits the data well, and follows λ^2 distribution with degree of freedom under the null hypothesis of independence. The DOF = $(r - 1)$ $(c - 1)$. r = row numbers and c = Columns numbers.

Example: In a matched case– control study, investigator collected data to assess the relationship existing between the use of kerosene lamp in the house and lung cancer. Control groups were matched with case with reference to age, smoking habit and sex. Verify the level of association between the use of kerosene lamp and Lung cancer.

Case (LUNG CANCER)		CONTROL (NO LUNG CANCER)		
		KEROSINE LAMP	NO KEROSINE LAMP	Total
	KEROSINE LAMP	35 -a	40 - b	75
	NO KEROSINE LAMP	10- c	115 -d	125
	Total	45	155	200

Solution:

$$OR = 10.0625$$

$$E_{11} = \frac{(45)(75)}{200} = 15.875,$$

$$E_{12} = \frac{(75)(155)}{200} = 58.125$$

$$E_{21} = \frac{(45)(125)}{200} = 28.125$$

$$E_{22} = \frac{(155)(125)}{200} = 96.875$$

O	E	(O-E)	(O-E)^2	(O-E)^2/E
35	16.875	18.125	328.5156	19.47
40	58.125	-18.125	328.5156	5.65
10	28.125	-18.125	328.5156	11.68
115	96.875	18.125	328.5156	3.39
				Σ(O-E)^2/E = 40.19

$$DOF = (r-1)(C-1) = (2-1)(2-1) = 1$$

$$\lambda^2_{cal} = 40.19$$

In case of matching pair the OR = B/C = 40/10 = 4

The $\quad \lambda^2_{cal} = \dfrac{(|B-C|-1)^2}{B+C} = \dfrac{(|40-10|-1)^2}{40+10} = 16.41$

The calculated value is greater than the standard value, hence the difference is significant, H_0 is rejected and this indicates that there is strong association between lamp using and lung cancer

Confidence interval at 95% level of significance for this OR is

$$Ln(OR) = \ln(OR) \pm 1.96 \times \sqrt{\frac{1}{40} + \frac{1}{10}}$$

$$= \ln(4) - 1.96 \times \sqrt{\frac{1}{40} + \frac{1}{10}} \quad \text{and} \quad \ln(4) + 1.96 \times \sqrt{\frac{1}{40} + \frac{1}{10}}$$

$$= 0.69 \text{ and } 2.08$$

Take exp for the values of ln(OR)

$$CI \text{ is } e^{0.69} \text{ and } e^{2.08}$$

$$(L, U) = (2.00, 8.00)$$

Continuity Corrections

The Chi-Square test is only approximate test. In case of 2×2 Contingency table the risk factor and Outcome variable must be discrete. Here the probability distribution is used to test the continuity of the data. In order to improve the continuous approximation to a discrete distribution, Yate's correction method is used, that will reduce the absolute difference between the observed and expected values in chi-square test.

The λ^2 can be obtained by the equation $\Sigma(|O-E|-1/2)^2 / E$ and for 2×2 tables it can be

written as $\dfrac{n\left(|ad-bc| - \dfrac{1}{2}n\right)^2}{(a+b)(c+d)(a+c)(b+d)}$, the $|O-E|$ and $|ad-bc|$ denotes absolute value of differences.

For the proportional value also Yates's correction can be applied and the equation can be written as

$$\frac{|p_1 - p_1| - \dfrac{1}{2}\left(\dfrac{1}{n_1} + \dfrac{1}{n_2}\right)}{\sqrt{p_c(1-p_c)}\left(\dfrac{1}{n_1} + \dfrac{1}{n_2}\right)}$$

$$P_c = \frac{n_1 p_1 + n_2 p_2}{n_1 + n_2}$$

Correlation

Correlation refers to the relationship between the variables. Some relationship found in certain type of variables, for example the measure of relationship between time interval and concentration of drug that distributes in the body.

"WHEN THE RELATIONSHIP IS OF QUANTITATIVE IN NATURE, THE APPROPRIATE STATISTICAL TOOL FOR DISCOVERING AND MEASURING THE RELATIONSHIP AND EXPRESSING IT IN A BRIEF FROMULA IS KNOWN AS CORRELATION".

Two variables are said to be correlated, if the change in one variable results in a corresponding change in the other variables.

Correlation is a statistical technique which measures and analyzes the degree or extent to which two variables or phenomenon fluctuates with reference to each other. The correlation also denotes the interdependence between two variables.

Correlation methods are used to measure the association between two or more variables. Here one will be concerned with observations for each sampling unit. Here investigator will be interested in finding, if two values are related, in the sense that one variable may be predicted from a knowledge of the other. Better is the prediction, the better is the correlation.

Degree of Correlation

The intensity of relationship between two variables can be ascertained by the quantitative value of coefficient of correlation which can be found out by computation.

Perfect Correlation

When changes between two variables are exactly proportional, there is perfect correlation between them. If the proportion of changes is in the same direction, then there is perfect positive correlation between two sets of variables. If equal proportional changes are in the opposite direction, then there is perfect negative correlation.

Absence of Correlation

If interdependence between the two variables does not exists, then it refers, the absence of correlation between the variables.

Karl Pearson has contributed an equation for measuring correlation. The result of that value will be denoted by r, that varies between ±1.

In case of Perfect +ve correlation, the value of r will be +1 and in case of Perfect negative correlation r will be -1.

If r is ± 0.9, this indicates that there is high degree correlation between two variables.

In Epidemiological study evidence can only show that the risk factor which is associated (correlated) with a higher incidence of disease in the population which is exposed to that risk factor. By measuring the coefficient of correlation, one can predict what is the intensity or degree of relationship between the exposure and outcome event. If the coefficient of correlation is very high, that is an indication to say that there is a good association between the exposure and outcome event.

Karl Pearson's Coefficient of Correlation (Covariance Method)

The correlation coefficient is a quantitative measure of the relationship of two variables. This will measure the intensity of linear relationship between two variables. This method was designed by Karl Pearson. This is the most widely used method to measure the relationship between two variables.

If X and Y are two variables, then the relationship between them is denoted by the symbol or notation r_{xy} or r.

The equation is

$\Sigma d_x d_y$ = Covariance of X & Y

σ_x = Standard deviation of X- series

σ_y = Standard deviation of Y- series

N = Number of subjects or items of both the series

Example 1: Compute the coefficient of correlation Age and Bilirubin level of 10 patients for the data listed below

AGE X	Bilirubin (mg/dl) Y	$d_x = (X - \bar{X})$	$d_y = (Y - \bar{Y})$	d^2_x	d^2_y	$d_x \times d_y$
70	11	12.4	1.71	153.76	2.92	21.204
68	12.3	10.4	3.01	108.16	9.06	31.304
81	14.7	23.4	5.41	547.56	29.27	126.594
59	9.1	1.4	−0.19	1.96	0.04	−0.266
64	7.8	6.4	−1.49	40.96	2.22	-9.536
48	6	−9.6	−3.29	92.16	10.82	31.584

Contd...

50	9	−7.6	−0.29	57.76	0.08	2.204
44	7	−13.6	−2.29	184.96	5.24	31.144
50	8	−7.6	−1.29	57.76	1.66	9.804
42	8	−15.6	−1.29	243.36	1.66	20.124
ΣX	ΣY			Σd^2_x	Σd^2_y	$\Sigma d_x \times d_y$
576	92.9			1488.4	62.989	264.16

$$\overline{X} = \frac{\Sigma X}{N} = \frac{576}{10} = 57.6 \qquad \overline{Y} = \frac{\Sigma Y}{N} = \frac{92.9}{10} = 9.29$$

$$\sigma_x = \sqrt{\frac{d^2_x}{N}} = \sqrt{\frac{1488.4}{10}} = 12.20 \qquad \sigma_y = \sqrt{\frac{d^2_y}{N}} = \sqrt{\frac{62.989}{10}} = 2.509$$

$$r = \frac{\Sigma d_x d_y}{N \sigma_x \sigma_y} = \frac{264.16}{10 \times 12.2 \times 2.509} = 0.863$$

Estimation of Confidence interval for coefficient of correlation: Fisher has designed a method for testing the significance between two coefficient of correlation. Here the coefficient of correlation r is transformed into Z, then it is named as Z-transformation.

The Z-Statistics is used to test, whether

(a) The observed value of r significantly differs at 5% level of significance or not

(b) To verify the level of significance between coefficients of correlation between two samples.

The equation used to transfer r into Z is

$$Z = \frac{1}{2} \ln\left(\frac{1+r}{1-r}\right) \quad \text{or} \quad Z = 1.1513 \log_{10}\left(\frac{1+r}{1-r}\right)$$

In this method the variance of Z is obtained by the equation $Var(Z) = \dfrac{1}{N-3}$, then the standard error of Z is $SE = \sqrt{\dfrac{1}{N-3}}$

Similarly ρ (population correlation coefficient) can be transformed into Z and that can be written as $\xi = \dfrac{1}{2} \ln\left(\dfrac{1+\rho}{1-\rho}\right)$ or $\xi = 1.1513 \log_{10}\left(\dfrac{1+\rho}{1-\rho}\right)$

The tests of significance can be done using the equation $\dfrac{Z - \xi}{SE}$

If the test value is .> 2.58, then the difference is significant at 1% level of significance.

Similarly if it is > 1.96, then the difference is significant at 5% level of significance and if it is > 3 then definitely the difference is significant.

Then the 95% confidence interval (r_L, r_U) of the coefficient of correlation r can be obtained by transforming the end points as

$$Z_L = Z - 1.96SE \text{ and } Z_U = Z + 1.95 \text{ SE}$$

Then the lower interval r_L is obtained by the equation $r_L = \dfrac{\text{Exp}(2Z_L)-1}{\text{Exp}(2Z_L)+1}$

Similarly the Upper interval is obtained by the equation $r_U = \dfrac{\text{Exp}(2Z_U)-1}{\text{Exp}(2Z_U)+1}$

CHAPTER 7

Regression Analysis

Correlation describes the strength of an association between two variables, and is completely symmetrical, the correlation between X and Y is the same as the correlation between Y and X. However, if the two variables are related it means that when one changes by a certain amount the other changes on an average by a certain amount. If Y represents the dependent variable and X the independent variable, this relationship is described as the regression of y on x.

The relationship can be represented in a simple equation is called the regression equation. In this context "regression" (the term is a historical anomaly) simply means that the average value of Y is a "function" of X, that is, Y changes when there is change in X.

Regression means to revert or return back. This term was first elucidated by English scientist Sir Francis Galton in 1877 also he was a British Biometrician.

But today the word regression is used in statistics has a much wider perspective without any reference to Biometry.

In general sense, the regression analysis means the estimation or prediction of one unknown value of one variable from the known value of the other variable. It is one of the most important statistical tools used in epidemiological study to measure association between resultant variable and exposure variable to analyze the data of clinical trial problems.

Regression analysis is one type of modeling technique used in epidemiological research to assess the relationships amongst a set of variables. Objective is to predict response or outcome from a set of explanatory variables.

Regression Analysis also is a mathematical measure of the average relationship between two or more variables in term of the original unit of data.

Simple linear regression analysis is a statistical technique that defines the functional relationship between two variables X and Y by the best fitting straight line. The straight is described by the equation $Y = \alpha + \beta X$. Here Y is considered as dependent variable (ordinate) and X is independent variable (abscissa), and α and β are the y-intercept and slope of the regression line.

Generally simple regression model will be written as $Y = \alpha + \beta X + \varepsilon$, where α and β are parameters and ε is named as random error. This technique is commonly used to:

1. To establish the functional relationship between optical density against drug concentration.
2. When the functional form of a response is unknown, but here one wish to represent a trend or rate as characterized by the slope.
3. When a process is described by relatively simple equation, that will establish a relation of response Y to a fixed value of X.

Formation of Simple Regression Equation by Matrix Method

Example:

$$
\begin{array}{cc}
X & Y \\
5 & 3 \\
8 & 4 \\
7 & 5 \\
6 & 2 \\
4 & 1
\end{array}
$$

$$
X = \begin{bmatrix} 1 & 5 \\ 1 & 8 \\ 1 & 7 \\ 1 & 6 \\ 1 & 4 \end{bmatrix}
\ Y = \begin{bmatrix} 3 \\ 4 \\ 5 \\ 2 \\ 1 \end{bmatrix}
\ \text{and} \ \alpha = \begin{bmatrix} a \\ b \end{bmatrix}
$$

$$
X^T = \begin{bmatrix} 1 & 1 & 1 & 1 & 1 \\ 5 & 8 & 7 & 6 & 4 \end{bmatrix}
$$

$$
X^T X = \begin{bmatrix} 1 & 1 & 1 & 1 & 1 \\ 5 & 8 & 7 & 6 & 4 \end{bmatrix}
\begin{bmatrix} 1 & 5 \\ 1 & 8 \\ 1 & 7 \\ 1 & 6 \\ 1 & 4 \end{bmatrix}
$$

$$
= \begin{bmatrix} 1+1+1+1+1 & 5+8+7+6+4 \\ 5+8+7+6+4 & 25+64+49+36+16 \end{bmatrix}
$$

$$
X^T X = \begin{bmatrix} 5 & 30 \\ 30 & 190 \end{bmatrix}
$$

Find Co-factor Matrix of $X^T X$

$$
\left.\begin{array}{l}
\text{Cofactor of } 5 = +(190) \\
\text{Cofactor of } 30 = -(30)
\end{array}\right\} - \text{First row elements}
$$

$$
\left.\begin{array}{l}
\text{Cofactor of } 30 = -(30) \\
\text{Cofactor of } 190 = +(5)
\end{array}\right\} - \text{Second row elements}
$$

$$
\text{Cofactor Matrix } X^T X = \begin{bmatrix} 190 & -30 \\ -30 & 5 \end{bmatrix}
$$

$$\text{adjoint}\left(X^{T}X\right) = \begin{bmatrix} 190 & -30 \\ -30 & 5 \end{bmatrix} \text{(Transpose of Co-factor Matrix)}$$

$$\left|X^{T}X\right| = \begin{bmatrix} 5 & 30 \\ 30 & 190 \end{bmatrix} = 950 - 900 = 50$$

$$\left[X^{T}X\right]^{-1} = \frac{1}{\left|X^{T}X\right|} \text{ adjoint } (X^{T} X)$$

$$= \frac{1}{50}\begin{bmatrix} 190 & -30 \\ -30 & 5 \end{bmatrix}$$

Find the product of $\quad X^{T}Y = \begin{bmatrix} 1 & 1 & 1 & 1 & 1 \\ 5 & 8 & 7 & 6 & 4 \end{bmatrix}\begin{bmatrix} 3 \\ 4 \\ 5 \\ 2 \\ 1 \end{bmatrix}$

$$= \begin{bmatrix} 3+4+5+2+1 \\ 5+8+7+6+4 \end{bmatrix}$$

$$= \begin{bmatrix} 15 \\ 98 \end{bmatrix}$$

Find the product of $\quad [X^{T} X]^{-1} \, X^{T}Y = \alpha = \begin{bmatrix} a \\ b \end{bmatrix}$

$$\begin{bmatrix} a \\ b \end{bmatrix} = \frac{1}{50}\begin{bmatrix} 190 & -30 \\ -30 & 5 \end{bmatrix}\begin{bmatrix} 15 \\ 98 \end{bmatrix}$$

$$= \frac{1}{50}\begin{bmatrix} 2850 - 2940 \\ -450 + 490 \end{bmatrix}$$

$$= \frac{1}{50}\begin{bmatrix} -90 \\ 40 \end{bmatrix}$$

$$\begin{bmatrix} a \\ b \end{bmatrix} = \begin{bmatrix} -1.8 \\ 0.8 \end{bmatrix}$$

$$a = -1.8, b = 0.8, \ Y = a + bX, \ Y = -1.8 + 0.8X$$

Methods of Least square to Form the regression Equation:

X	Y
5	3
8	4
7	5
6	2
4	1

Solution:

x	y	$dx=(x-\bar{x})$	$dy=(y-\bar{y})$	dx^2	dy^2	dxdy
5	3	−1	0	1	0	0
8	4	2	1	4	1	2
7	5	1	2	1	4	2
6	2	0	−1	0	1	0
4	1	−2	−2	4	4	4

$Sxx = \sum dx^2 = 10$ $Syy = \sum dy^2 = 10$ $Sxy = \sum dxdy = 8$

$\sum x = 30$ $\sum y = 15$

$\bar{x} = \sum x / n$ $\bar{y} = \sum y / n$

$= 30/5 = 6$ $= 15/5 = 3$

$$b = \frac{sxy}{sxx} = 8/10 = 0.8$$

$$a = \bar{y} - b \times \bar{x}$$

$$a = 3 - 0.8 \times 6$$

$$a = -1.8$$

Anova Table for Simple Linear Regression

Sources of Variation	Sum of squares	Degree of freedom	Mean Squares	F ratio
Variation due to regression	$SS_r = \dfrac{S_{xy}^2}{S_{xx}}$	DOF=1	$MSS_r = \dfrac{SS_r}{dof}$	$MSS_r / MSSe$
Due to Error	$SS_e = S_{yy} - \dfrac{S_{xy}^2}{S_{xx}}$	$n - 2$	$MSSe = \dfrac{SS_e}{dof}$	

Sources of Variation	Sum of squares	Degree of freedom	Mean Squares	F ratio
Variation due to regression	$SS_r = \dfrac{8^2}{10} = 6.4$	DOF=1	$MSS_r = \dfrac{6.4}{1} = 6.4$	$MSS_r / MSSe$
Due to Error	$SS_e = 10 - 6.4 = 3.6$	$n - 2 = 5 - 2 = 3$	$MSSe = \dfrac{3.6}{3} = 1.3$	$=6.4/1.3 = 4.92$
Total	$Syy = 10$	$N - 1 = 4$		

For degree of freedom $\lambda_{nr} = 1$ and $\lambda_{dr} = 3$, the standard value of F = 17.4. Then the difference is not significant. This indicates that x has no role or effect in predicting the dependent variable y.

Example 2: The data given in the table is about the pulmonary anatomical dead space (in ml) and height (in cm) of 15 children. Find the coefficient correlation between height and anatomical dead space and form the simple regression equation to establish the functional relationship between height and anatomical dead space

Patient No.	1	2	3	4	5	6	7	8	9	10	11	12	13	14	15
Height	110	116	124	129	131	138	142	150	153	155	156	159	164	168	174
Dead Space (ml)-Y	44	31	43	45	56	79	57	56	58	92	78	64	88	112	101

Solution:

Child Age	X	Y	dx= $(X-\overline{X})$	dy= $(Y-\overline{Y})$	dx^2	dy^2	dxdy
1	1	112	43	−32.6	−23.67	1062.76	560.2689
2	2	115	32	−29.6	−34.67	876.16	1202.009
3	3	123	44	−21.6	−22.67	466.56	513.9289
4	4	127	46	−17.6	−20.67	309.76	427.2489
5	5	131	55	−13.6	−11.67	184.96	136.1889
6	6	135	78	−9.6	11.33	92.16	128.3689
7	7	142	59	−2.6	−7.67	6.76	58.8289
8	8	152	52	7.4	−14.67	54.76	215.2089
9	9	153	59	8.4	−7.67	70.56	58.8289
10	10	155	90	10.4	23.33	108.16	544.2889
11	11	156	77	11.4	10.33	129.96	106.7089
12	12	158	65	13.4	−1.67	179.56	2.7889
13	13	165	90	20.4	23.33	416.16	544.2889
14	14	168	110	23.4	43.33	547.56	1877.489
15	15	175	100	30.4	33.33	924.16	1110.889
N= 15	$\sum X = 2167$	$\sum Y = 1000$			$\sum dx^2$ =5430.00	$\sum dy^2$ =7487.334	$\sum dxdy$ =5329.34

$$\overline{X} = \frac{\sum X}{N} \qquad \overline{Y} = \frac{\sum Y}{N}$$
$$= 2167/15 \qquad =1000/15$$
$$= 144.47 \qquad =66.67$$

$$sd(X) = \sqrt{\frac{\sum dx^2}{N}} = \sqrt{\frac{5430}{15}} = 19.03$$

$$sd(Y) = \sqrt{\frac{\Sigma dy^2}{N}} = \sqrt{\frac{7487.334}{15}} = 22.34$$

$$r = \frac{\Sigma dxdy}{N \times sd(X) \times sd(Y)} = 5329.34 / (15 \times 19.03 \times 22.34) = 0.85$$

Formation of Regression equation:

$$b = \frac{\Sigma dxdy}{\Sigma dx^2} = 5329.34 / 5430.00 = 0.99$$

$$a = \overline{Y} - b \times \overline{X} = 66.67 - 0.99 \times 144.47 = -76.73$$

Regression Equation is $Y = -76.73 + 0.99x$

Graph between Height and observed value of anatomical dead space

(Anatomic dead space is the total volume of the conducting airways from the nose or mouth down to the level of the terminal bronchioles and is about **150 ml** on the average in humans. The anatomic dead space fills with inspired air at the end of each inspiration, but this air is exhaled unchanged.)

Age	X	Y Observed Values	$Y1 = -76.73 + 0.99 \times X$ Predicted Values
1	112	43	34.15
2	115	32	37.12
3	123	44	45.04
4	127	46	49
5	131	55	52.96
6	135	78	56.92
7	142	59	63.85
8	152	52	73.75
9	153	59	74.74
10	155	90	76.72
11	156	77	77.71
12	158	65	79.69
13	165	90	86.62
14	168	110	89.59
15	175	100	96.52

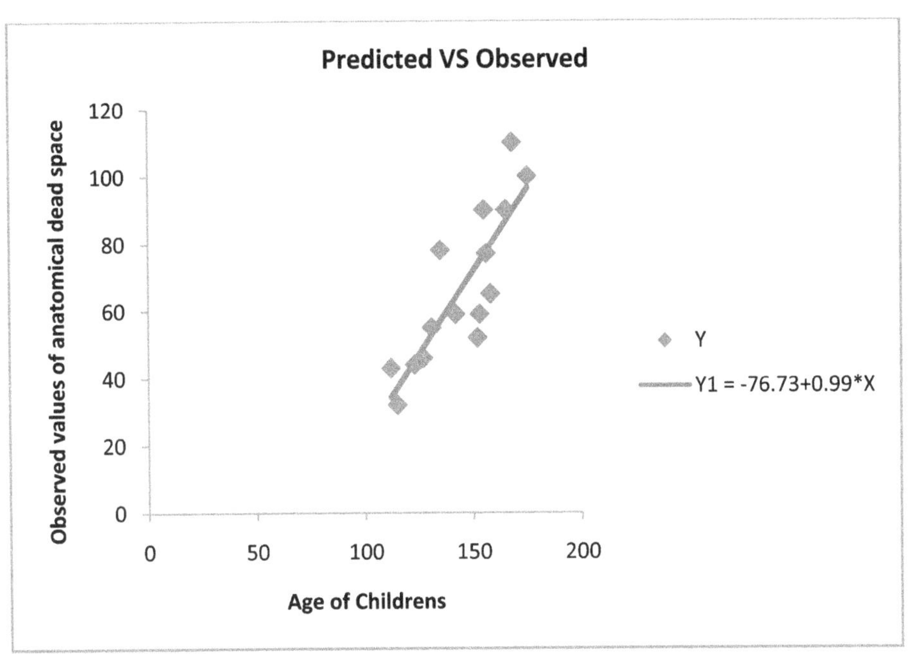

Performing Regression Analysis to verify the level of significance (ANOVA)

Age	X	Y	$Y^1 = -76.73+0.99 \times X$	$(Y - \overline{Y})^2$	$(Y^1 - \overline{Y})^2$
1	112	43	34.15	560.2689	1057.5504
2	115	32	37.12	1202.0089	873.2025
3	123	44	45.04	513.9289	467.8569
4	127	46	49	427.2489	312.2289
5	131	55	52.96	136.1889	187.9641
6	135	78	56.92	128.3689	95.0625
7	142	59	63.85	58.8289	7.9524
8	152	52	73.75	215.2089	50.1264
9	153	59	74.74	58.8289	65.1249
10	155	90	76.72	544.2889	101.0025
11	156	77	77.71	106.7089	121.8816
12	158	65	79.69	2.7889	169.5204
13	165	90	86.62	544.2889	398.0025
14	168	110	89.59	1877.4889	525.3264
15	175	100	96.52	1110.8889	891.0225
				SST= 7487.3335	SSR =5323.8249

SST = Total Sum Squares, SSR = Sum of the squares due regression

SSE = Residual Error = SST − SSR = 7487.3335 − 5323.8249 = 2163.5086,

ANOVA[a]

	Model	Sum of Squares	df	Mean Square	F	Sig.
1	Regression	5323.8249	1	5323.8249	31.99	.00001 < 0.05
	Residual	2163.5086	13	166.424		
	Total	7487.3335	14			

a. Dependent Variable: Dead Space
b. Predictors: (Constant), Height

Data is analyzed using SPSS 22 to verify the level of significance using experimental or observed data.

Model Summary

Model	R	R Square	Adjusted R Square	Std. Error of the Estimate
1	.845[a]	.714	.692	12.82455

a. Predictors: (Constant), Height

ANOVA

	Model	Sum of Squares	df	Mean Square	F	Sig.
1.	Regression	5349.234	1	5349.234	32.5 24	.0000 <0.05
	Residual	2138.099	13	164.469		
	Total	7487.333	14			

a. Dependent Variable: Dead Space
b. Predictors: (Constant), Height

Coefficients

	Model	Unstandardized Coefficients		Standardized Coefficients	t	Sig.
		B	Std. Error	Beta		
1.	(Constant)	−76.725	25.360		-3.025	.010
	Height	.993	.174	.845	5.703	.000

a. Dependent Variable: Dead Space

In SPSS Software three decimal are considered, due that there is slight difference between calculated value using excel and SPSS, but SST remains s same in both cases.

Example: The data given below is about the number of deaths in 15 cities due to the exposure of mean atmospheric smoke (x_1 in mg/m) and mean atmospheric sulfur dioxide content (x_2, in ppm). Perform regression analysis and verify the effect of these two factors and compute F-distribution value and verify the level of significance at 5% and 1% level.

X_1	X_2	Y
1.2	1.2	112
0.49	0.16	141
0.7	0.23	142
1.2	0.14	130
2.64	0.75	190
3.45	0.86	290
4.45	1.34	512
4.46	1.34	513
1.22	0.47	420
1.22	0.47	270

Solution:

X_1	X_2	Y	$x_1 =$ $(X_1-\overline{X1})$	$x_2 =$ $(X_2-\overline{X2})$	$y =$ $(Y-\overline{Y})$	x_1^2	x_2^2	x_1y	x_2y	x_1x_2
1.2	1.2	112	-0.9	0.5	-160	0.81	0.25	144	-80	-0.45
0.49	0.16	141	-1.61	-0.54	-131	2.5921	0.2916	210.91	70.74	0.8694
0.7	0.23	142	-1.4	-0.47	-130	1.96	0.2209	182	61.1	0.658
1.2	0.14	130	-0.9	-0.56	-142	0.81	0.3136	127.8	79.52	0.504
2.64	0.75	190	0.54	0.05	-82	0.2916	0.0025	-44.28	-4.1	0.027
3.45	0.86	290	1.35	0.16	18	1.8225	0.0256	24.3	2.88	0.216
4.45	1.34	512	2.35	0.64	240	5.5225	0.4096	564	153.6	1.504
4.46	1.34	513	2.36	0.64	241	5.5696	0.4096	568.76	154.24	1.5104
1.22	0.47	420	-0.88	-0.23	148	0.7744	0.0529	-130.24	-34.04	0.2024
1.22	0.47	270	-0.88	-0.23	-2	0.7744	0.0529	1.76	0.46	0.2024
$\sum X_1 =$ 21.03	$\sum X_2$ =6.96	$\sum Y$ =2720				$\sum x_1^2$ =20.9271	$\sum x_2^2$ =2.0292	$\sum x_1y$ = 1649.01	$\sum x_2y$ =404.4	$\sum x_1x_2$ = 5.2436
$\overline{X1}$ =2.10	$\overline{X2}=$ 0.70	$\overline{Y}=$ 272								

$$b_1 = \frac{\left(x_2^2\right)\left(\Sigma x_1y\right) - \Sigma\left(x_1x_2\right)\left(x_2y\right)}{\left(\Sigma x_1^2\right)\left(\Sigma x_2^2\right) - \left(\Sigma x_1x_2\right)^2}$$

b1 = 81.87

$$b_2 = \frac{\left(x_1^2\right)\left(\Sigma x_2 y\right) - \Sigma\left(x_1 x_2\right)\left(x_1 y\right)}{\left(\Sigma x_1^2\right)\left(\Sigma x_2^2\right) - \left(\Sigma x_1 x_2\right)^2}$$

$$b_2 = -12.28$$

$$a = \overline{Y} - b_1 \overline{X1} - b_2 \overline{X2} = 272 - 81 \times 2.10 - (12.28) \times 0.70 = 108.37$$

Then the regression equation is $Y = a + b_1 X_1 + b_2 X_2 = 108.37 + 81.87 X_1 - 12.28 X_2$

The data is analyzed using SPSS – 22 and summary of the result is as listed below.

X_1	X_2	Y	$Y^1 = 108.37 + 81.87 X_1 - 12.28 X_2$	$(Y\text{-Mean}(Y))^2$	$(Y^1\text{-Mean}(Y))^2$
1.2	1.2	112	191.878	25600	6419.53
0.49	0.16	141	146.5215	17161	15744.85
0.7	0.23	142	162.8546	16900	11912.72
1.2	0.14	130	204.8948	20164	4503.11
2.64	0.75	190	315.2968	6724	1874.61
3.45	0.86	290	380.2607	324	11720.38
4.45	1.34	512	456.2363	57600	33943.01
4.46	1.34	513	457.055	58081	34245.35
1.22	0.47	420	202.4798	21904	4833.06
1.22	0.47	270	202.4798	4	4833.06
		Mean(Y) = 272		SST = 224462	SSR = 130029.69

ANOVA

Model	Sum of Squares	df	Mean Square	F	Sig.
Regression	SSR = 130047.144	K-1 = 3 – 1 = 2	65023.572	4.821	.048[b]
Residual	SSE = 94414.856	N- K = 10 – 3 = 7	13487.837		
Total	SST = 224462.000	N- 1 = 10 – 1 = 9			

The data is analyzed using SPSS – 22 and summary of the result is as listed below.

Model Summary

Model	R	R Square	Adjusted R Square	Std. Error of the Estimate
1	.761[a]	.579	.459	116.13715

a. Predictors: (Constant), X2, X1

ANOVA[a]

Model		Sum of Squares	df	Mean Square	F	Sig.
1	Regression	130047.144	2	65023.572	4.821	.048[b]
	Residual	94414.856	7	13487.837		
	Total	224462.000	9			

a. Dependent Variable: Y

b. Predictors: (Constant), X2, X1

Coefficients[a]

Model		Un-standardized Coefficients		Standardized Coefficients	t	Sig.
		B	Std. Error	Beta		
1	(Constant)	a=108.367	68.835		1.574	.159
	X1	b1=81.880	42.764	.791	1.915	.097
	X2	b2=-12.300	137.336	-.037	-.090	.931

a. Dependent Variable: Y

Association Versus Prediction model in Epidemiology

In epidemiological study there are two models, which are commonly used are 'Association model' and a 'Prediction model'.

In case of 'Association model' very often epidemiologists use the regression model, where they identify an exposure variable of interest (say X) and looks its relationship with the outcome variable (say Y). Other independent variables (say $Z1, Z2, Z3,…$) are simply moderators of the effect of X or not. If yes, the interaction term and the main effect are included in the model. If not, we ignore the interaction term and further evaluate whether the independent variable is a confounder or not. Accordingly, we decide whether main effect is to be included or not to be included in the final or reduced model.

In the 'Prediction model', investigator would like to verify how model fits the given data and explains the outcome variable (Y). All the independent variables will be taken as $X1, X2, X3$, and if there is any interaction between the variables, they can be written as $X1{\times}X2, X1{\times}X3, X2{\times}X3$. Then the models are evaluated for goodness-of-fit, R-square or predictive ability using different validation techniques called regression diagnostics.

Regression Diagnostics

Whenever a particular model is selected there the investigator need to assess how well the data will fit in the model, or how much the predicted values are close to the experimental values. Deviations of predicted values from observed values must be normal. The statistical test which assesses model to verify how the data fit is known as "Goodness-of-fit statistics". Here the investigator hopes that the model fits the data adequately and statistical test which is applied to analyze the experimental data must be significant.

While goodness-of-fit statistics tell us how well a particular model fits the data, but they tell us a little about the lack of fit, or why and where a particular model fails to fit the data.

Regression diagnostics primarily focus on methods for analyzing residuals, assessing the influence of outliers and assessing problem of collinearity (i.e. inter-relationship between two independent variables or predictors).

After performing experiment, the investigator needs to understand that the selected mathematical models need not always be able to explain all the variation in the observed data. Statistical modeling techniques using maximum likelihood estimation (MLE) or weighted least squares (WLS) are often employed to describe variation in terms of a parsimonious model.

Steps to be observed in regression analysis: The study of relationships between variables and the generation of risk scores are very important elements of medical research. The proper performance of regression analysis requires that a few important factors should be considered and tested.

Relationship between Variables

Before a regression analysis is performed, the causal relationships among the variables to be considered must be examined from the point of view of their content and/or temporal relationship. The fact that an independent variable turns out to be significant says nothing about causality. This is an especially relevant point with respect to observational studies.

Sample size Planning for regression analysis: The number of cases needed for a regression analysis depends on the number of independent variables and of their expected effects (strength of relationships). If the sample is too small, only very strong relationships will be demonstrable. The sample size can be planned in the light of the researchers' expectations regarding the coefficient of determination (r^2) and the regression coefficient (b). Furthermore, at least 20 times as many observations should be made as there are independent variables to be studied; thus, if one wants to study 2 independent variables, one should make at least 40 observations.

Missing Values of Experimental Result

Missing values are a common problem in medical data. Whenever the value of either a dependent or an independent variable is missing, that particular observed data has to be excluded from the group before performing regression analysis. If many values are missing from the dataset, the effective sample size will be appreciably diminished, and the sample may then turn out to be too small to yield significant findings, despite of advance planning. In this situation investigator should plan for large sample size, to overcome this problem.

Selection of data Sample

A further important point to be considered is the composition of the study population. If there are subpopulations within it that behave differently with respect to the independent variables in question, then a real effect (or the lack of an effect) may be masked from the analysis and remain undetected. Suppose, when an investigator wants to study the effect of sex on weight, the population selected for study which consists half of children under age 6 and the remaining half are adults. Linear regression analysis over the entire population reveals an effect of sex on weight. In that case, a subgroup analysis is performed in which children and adults are separated into two groups, then the effect of sex on weight is seen only in adults. This type of analysis has to be performed when the subgroups have been predefined, and the questions already formulated, before the data analysis begins; furthermore, multiple testing should be taken into account.

Selection of variable based on interaction between the independent variables.

If an investigator considers multiple independent variables in a multivariable regression, some of them may be interdependent. An independent variable that would be found to have a strong effect in a univariate regression model might not turn out to have any appreciable effect in a multivariable regression with variable selection. This will happen if this particular variable itself depends so strongly on the other independent variables that it makes no additional contribution towards explaining the dependent variable. In this situation investigator should observe the interrelationship between the variables at the time of analyzing the experimental result and drawing the conclusion about the data.

Confidence Interval for Slope (b) and Intercept (a)

To construct a confidence interval for slope – b the standard error of b, $S_b = \dfrac{Syx}{\sqrt{\Sigma\left(X-\overline{X}\right)^2}}$ is estimated and t- is estimated using equation $t = \dfrac{b-0}{S_b}$.

The value of t for degree of freedom N – K at the level of significance (95% or 99%) will be compared with calculated value (computed value) of t. If the computed value of t is greater than the table value, the relationship will be linear with the computed value of standard error, then the confidence limits of b can be obtained using the equation $b \pm 1.96 S_b$ at 95% level of significance for the corresponding degree of freedom (N – K)

Similarly, the confidence interval for a also can obtained by the equation is a ± 1.96

$$Sb \sqrt{\frac{1}{N} + \frac{\overline{X^2}}{\Sigma\left(X-\overline{X}\right)^2}}$$

Problem:

X	Y	dx= (X-Mean(x))	dy= (Y-Mean(y))	dx^2	dy^2	dx×dy	$y^1=$ 7.6×x +32	$(y-y^1)$	$(y-y^1)^2$
3	40	-2	-30	4	900	60	54.8	-14.8	219.04
3	55	-2	-15	4	225	30	54.8	0.2	0.04
4	55	-1	-15	1	225	15	62.4	-7.4	54.76
4	60	-1	-10	1	100	10	62.4	-2.4	5.76
4	75	1	5	1	25	-5	62.4	12.6	158.76
5	70	0	0	0	0	0	70	0	0

X	Y	dx = (X-Mean(x))	dy = (Y-Mean(y))	dx^2	dy^2	dx×dy	y^1 = 7.6×x + 32	$(y-y^1)$	$(y-y^1)^2$
5	80	0	10	0	100	0	70	10	100
5	75	0	5	0	25	0	70	5	25
6	90	1	20	1	400	20	77.6	12.4	153.76
6	80	1	10	1	100	10	77.6	2.4	5.76
7	75	2	5	4	25	10	85.2	-10.2	104.04
8	85	3	15	9	225	45	92.8	-7.8	60.84
60	840			26	2350	195	840		887.76

$$\overline{X} = 5$$

$$\overline{Y} = 70$$

$$\sigma_x = 1.47$$

$$\sigma_y = 13.99$$

$$r = 0.8$$

Regression Equation Y on X

$$(Y - \overline{Y}) = \left(r \frac{\sigma x}{\sigma y}(X - \overline{X}) \right)$$

$$(Y - 70) = 0.8 \times 14/1.47(X - 5)$$

$$Y - 70 = 7.6X - 38.0$$

$$Y = 7.6X + 32$$

Standard Error of Estimate:

$$S_{yx} = \sqrt{\frac{(y - y^1)}{N - k}} = \sqrt{\frac{(887.76)}{12 - 2}} = 9.42$$

Standard error of b:

$$S_b = \frac{S_{yx}}{\sqrt{\Sigma(X - \overline{X})^2}} = \frac{9.42}{\sqrt{26}} = 1.85$$

$$t = \frac{b - 0}{S_b} = \frac{7.6 - 0}{1.85} = 4.1$$

The table value of t at 10 degree of freedom at 5% level of significance = 2.228, at 1% level of is 3.169. The calculated value of t = 4.1 > 3.169 and also 4.1 > 2.228, hence b differ significantly from 0, hence the relationship between X and Y is significant at 5% as well as at 1% level of significance.

Hence the value of b at 95% level of confidence (or 5% level of significance) b ± 1.96 × s_b = 7.6 ± 1.96 × 1.85 = 7.6 ± 3.626

The value of a at 95% level of confidence (or 5% level of significance) is a ± 1.96

$$S_{yx}\sqrt{\frac{1}{N}+\frac{\overline{X^2}}{\Sigma\left(X-\overline{X}\right)^2}}=32\pm1.96\times9.42\sqrt{\frac{1}{12}+\frac{5^2}{26}}$$

$$=32\pm1.96\times9.42\ 8\times1.02$$

$$=32\pm18.83$$

$$=13.17\text{-----}50.83$$

Multiple regression analysis using normal equation form: In statistics to perform statistical analysis we confined to the simultaneous study of two variables. But most of the studies in medical, Pharmaceutical and Biological science the value of one dependent variable or phenomenon of variable under consideration will be affected by multiple factors or variables, many of them may inter-related among themselves. To study and to predict the effect of these causal factors multiple regression is one of the important tools for studying the relationship between three or more variable.

For example, when we consider the body weight of an individual subject, which can be considered as a dependent variable, that will be depending on the independent variable like height and age of the individual subject.

When more than one dependent variable is included in a statistical model is called as multiple regression. Epidemiological and medical research investigator often apply multiple regression technique to measure or to evaluate association between the variables while adjusting for the potential confounding effect of other factor or variables. For example, in a study assessing the association between diet and blood pressure, age, sex and race were considered to be potential confounder.

To obtain the multiple regression equation minimum of two independent variables and one dependent variable are required.

The General form of the multiple regression can be written as

$Y = a+ b_1x_1 + b_2x_2 +\ldots\ldots..+b_nx_n + \varepsilon$, where b_1, b_2 …b_n are regression coefficients of the variables x_1, x_2,….x_n and b_0 is intercept.

If x_1 and x_2 are two independent variable and y is one dependent variable, then the regression coefficients and intercept can be obtained by the equations

$$Y= a + b_1x_1 + b_2x_2$$

$$b_1=\frac{\left(x_2^2\right)\left(\Sigma x_1y\right)-\Sigma\left(x_1x_2\right)\left(x_2y\right)}{\left(\Sigma x_1^2\right)\left(\Sigma x_2^2\right)-\left(\Sigma x_1x_2\right)^2}$$

$$b_2=\frac{\left(x_1^2\right)\left(\Sigma x_2y\right)-\Sigma\left(x_1x_2\right)\left(x_1y\right)}{\left(\Sigma x_1^2\right)\left(\Sigma x_2^2\right)-\left(\Sigma x_1x_2\right)^2}$$

Example:

X1	X2	Y	x1=(X1-Mean(X1)	x2= (X2-Mean(X2)	Y=(Y-Mean(Y))	$x1^2$	$x2^2$	x1Y	x2y	x1x2
10	36	40	-30	1	-20	900	1	600	-20	-30
20	33	45	-20	-2	-15	400	4	300	30	40
30	37	50	-10	2	-10	100	4	100	-20	-20
40	37	65	0	2	5	0	4	0	10	0
50	34	70	10	-1	10	100	1	100	-10	-10
60	32	70	20	-3	10	400	9	200	-30	-60
70	36	80	30	1	20	900	1	600	20	30
280	245	420				2800	24	1900	-20	-50
	Average of Y $\bar{Y}$= 420/7 =60									
N =7										
Mean(X1)= $\overline{X1}$ =280/7 = 40			b1	0.689						
Mean(X2)=$\overline{X2}$ = 245/7= 35			b2	0.603						
	a= $\bar{Y}$-b1$\overline{X1}$ - b2$\overline{X2}$ a=60 – 0.689*40 – 0.603*35			11.33						

X1	X2	Y	Y(pred) =11.33 + 0.689*X1 +0.603*X2	(Y - Mean(Y))^2	(Y(Pre)-Mean(Y))^2
10	36	40	39.928	400	402.89
20	33	45	45.009	225	224.73
30	37	50	54.311	100	32.36
40	37	65	61.201	25	1.44
50	34	70	66.282	100	39.46
60	32	70	71.966	100	143.19
70	36	80	81.268	400	452.33
		60		SST= 1350	SSR =1296.40

SSE = SST- SSR =1350 – 1296.40

Sources of Variation	Sum of Squares	DOF	Mean Squares	F-Distribution	P = 0.05	Remarks
Due to Regression(SSR)	SSR = 1296.40	K-1 = 3 – 1 = 2	MSR = SSR/K-1 = 1296/2 = 648.20	MSR/MSE = 48.36	0.0015<0.05	Difference is Significant
Due to Error(SSR	SSE = 53.63	N – K = 7 – 3 = 4	MSE = SSE/4 = 53.63 / 4 = 13.4			
TOtal	SST =1350	N- 1 = 6				

If the independent variables are three and one dependent variable, then the functional relational ship can be established using equation which are used calculate regression coefficients and the intercept

$$b_1 = \frac{\left(\Sigma x_2^2 \Sigma x_3^2 \Sigma x_1 y\right) - \left(\Sigma x_1 x_2 \Sigma x_1 x_3 \Sigma x_2 y \Sigma x_3 y\right)}{\left(\Sigma x_1^2 \Sigma x_3^2\right) - \left(\Sigma x_1 x_2\right)^2 \left(\Sigma x_1 x_3\right)^2 \left(\Sigma x_2 x_3\right)^2}$$

$$b_2 = \frac{\left(\Sigma x_1^2 \Sigma x_3^2 \Sigma x_2 y\right) - \left(\Sigma x_2 x_1 \Sigma x2 x_3 \Sigma x_1 y \Sigma x_3 y\right)}{\left(\Sigma x_1^2 \Sigma x_2^2 \Sigma x_3^2\right) - \left(\Sigma x_1 x_2\right)^2 \left(\Sigma x_1 x_3\right)^2 \left(\Sigma x_2 x_3\right)^2}$$

$$b_3 = \frac{\left(\Sigma x_1^2 \Sigma x_2^2 \Sigma x_3 y\right) - \left(\Sigma x_3 x_1 \Sigma x_3 x_2 \Sigma x_1 y \Sigma x_2 y\right)}{\left(\Sigma x_1^2 \Sigma x_2^2 \Sigma x_3^2\right) - \left(\Sigma x_1 x_2\right)^2 \left(\Sigma x_1 x_3\right)^2 \left(\Sigma x_2 x_3\right)^2}$$

$$a = \overline{Y} - b_1 \times \overline{X1} - b_2 \times \overline{X2} - b_3 \times \overline{X3}$$

X1	X2	X3	Y	x1 = (X1 - $\overline{X1}$)	x2 = (X2 - $\overline{X2}$)	x3 = (X3 - $\overline{X3}$)	y= (Y-$\overline{Y}$)	x1y	x2y	x3y	x1x2	x1x3	x2x3	x1^2	x2^2	x3^2
-1	-1	-1	23	-1	-1	-1	-8.6	8.6	8.6	8.6	1	1	1	1	1	1
1	-1	-1	27	1	-1	-1	-4.6	-4.6	4.6	4.6	-1	-1	1	1	1	1
-1	1	-1	24	-1	1	-1	-7.6	7.6	-7.6	7.6	-1	1	-1	1	1	1
1	1	-1	38	1	1	-1	6.4	6.4	6.4	-6.4	1	-1	-1	1	1	1
-1	-1	1	36	-1	-1	1	4.4	-4.4	-4.4	4.4	1	-1	-1	1	1	1
1	-1	1	34	1	-1	1	2.4	2.4	-2.4	2.4	-1	1	-1	1	1	1
-1	1	1	37	-1	1	1	5.4	-5.4	5.4	5.4	-1	-1	1	1	1	1
1	1	1	34	1	1	1	2.4	2.4	2.4	2.4	1	1	1	1	1	1
0	0	0	28	0	0	0	-3.6	0	0	0	0	0	0	0	0	0
0	0	0	35	0	0	0	3.4	0	0	0	0	0	0	0	0	0
ΣX1 =0	ΣX2= 0	ΣX3= 0	Σy = 316					Σx1y =13	Σx2 y= 13	Σx3y = 13	Σx1x2 = 0	Σx1x3 = 0	Σx2x3 = 0	Σx1^2 =8	Σx2^2 =8	Σx3^2 =8
$\overline{X1}$= 0	$\overline{X2}$ =0	$\overline{X3}$ = 0	$\overline{Y}$ =31.6													

$$b_1 = \frac{\left(\Sigma x_2^2 \Sigma x_3^2 \Sigma x_1 y\right) - \left(\Sigma x_1 x_2 \Sigma x_1 x_3 \Sigma x_2 y \Sigma x_3 y\right)}{\left(\Sigma x_1^2 \Sigma x_2^2 \Sigma x_3^2\right) - \left(\Sigma x_1 x_2\right)^2 \left(\Sigma x_1 x_3\right)^2 \left(\Sigma x_2 x_3\right)^2}$$

$$= (8 \times 8 \times 13) - (0 \times 0 \times 13 \times 13)/(8 \times 8 \times 8) - (0^2 \times 0^2 \times 0^2)$$

$$= 832/512 = 1.625$$

$$b_2 = \frac{\left(\Sigma x_1^2 \Sigma x_3^2 \Sigma x_2 y\right) - \left(\Sigma x_2 x_1 \Sigma x_2 x_3 \Sigma x_1 y \Sigma x_3 y\right)}{\left(\Sigma x_1^2 \Sigma x_2^2 \Sigma x_3^2\right) - \left(\Sigma x_1 x_2\right)^2 \left(\Sigma x_1 x_3\right)^2 \left(\Sigma x_2 x_3\right)^2}$$

$$= (8 \times 8 \times 13) - (0 \times 0 \times 13 \times 13)/(8 \times 8 \times 8) - (0^2 \times 0^2 \times 0^2)$$

$$= 832/512 = 1.625$$

$$b_3 = \frac{\left(\Sigma x_1^2 \Sigma x_2^2 \Sigma x_3 y\right) - \left(\Sigma x_3 x_1 \Sigma x_3 x_2 \Sigma x_1 y \Sigma x_2 y\right)}{\left(\Sigma x_1^2 \Sigma x_2^2 \Sigma x_3^2\right) - \left(\Sigma x_1 x_2\right)^2 \left(\Sigma x_1 x_3\right)^2 \left(\Sigma x_2 x_3\right)^2}$$

$$= (8 \times 8 \times 29) - (0 \times 0 \times 13 \times 13)/(8 \times 8 \times 8) - (0^2 \times 0^2 \times 0^2)$$

$$= 1856/512 = 3.625$$

Example:

$$a = \overline{Y} - b1 \times \overline{X1} - b2 \times \overline{X2} - b3 \times \overline{X3}$$
$$= 31.6 - 1.525 \times 0 - 1.625 \times 0 = 3.625 \times 0$$
$$a = 31.6$$
$$Y = a + b1\ X1 + b2X2 + b3X3$$
$$Y = 31.6 + 1.625X1 + 1.625X2 + 3.625X2$$

Example: The data listed below is about the investigation done by the researcher which will be measuring the association between body mass index (dependent Variable), sex age and diet score(independent variables) as per the type of food consumed by individual subjects who have been selected for study. Sex will be coded as 0 for female and 1 for male and age > 20 is coded as 1 and age < 20 is coded as 0. Construct multiple regression by matrix method and analyze the data to verify the level of significance.

Patient ID	Score of Diet	Sex	Age> 20	BMI
1	4	0	1	27
2	7	1	1	29
3	6	1	0	23
4	2	0	0	20
5	3	0	1	21

BMI = 18.0 + 1.5 (diet score) + 1.6 (Sex) + 4.2 age

Note that the numbers in red are the coefficients that the analysis provided.

CHAPTER 8

Sample Size Technique

Sample is the part of the population that helps us to draw inferences about the population. In research of Collecting the complete information about the population is not possible and it is time consuming and expensive. Thus, we need an appropriate sample size so that we can make inferences about the population based on that sample.

There is no certain rule of thumb to determine the sample size. Some researchers do, however, support a rule of thumb when using the sample size.

For example, many investigators say to perform regression analysis, they say that there should be at least 10 subjects or observations for different variables. If we consider three independent variables, then as per rule there should be 30 subjects in the study group.

Quality of clinical trials has improved steadily over last two decades, but certain areas in trial methodology still require special attention like in sample size calculation. The sample size is one of the basic steps in planning any clinical trial and any negligence in its calculation may lead to rejection of true findings and false results may get approval.

The determination of sample size is critical planning in clinical research, because sample size is usually the most important factor determining the time and funding necessary to perform the research. The sample has a profound impact on the likelihood of finding statistical significance.

Sample size n is one of the aspect that come to the mind of an investigator, when they are planning for an investigation. One of the most frequent problems in statistical analysis is the determination of the appropriate sample size. The sample size should be neither too large nor too small. When an investigator decides to go for very large sample size, that would waste the resources. If it is possible to get reliable answer for the experiment with only 200 subjects, then the investigator need not waste their time and money on resources to perform an experiment on 250 or more subjects.

A small sample size also may not give complete evidence, then the result obtained by doing study with that sample size may fail to achieve objective of the research. Again this is also is a waste of resources and time. In case some interventional studies, choosing very large sample is unethical, because some subjects are unnecessarily exposed to an intervention, when their utility is in doubt. Similarly, when the small sample size is used and subjects are exposed to an experiment, that is not going to give result or may not yield any result, is also waste of time and money.

According to the opinion of many statisticians, if the sample size is very large, the reliability of the result will be more appropriate. But in some situation, it becomes very difficult for an investigator to go for large sample size and it becomes burden for him/her. Similarly the sample size is smaller, investigator cannot take the decision, that the study will be useless.

In that situation investigator should consult the statistician, who will be able to able suggest an adequate sample size, which is required for their study, depending on the objective of the study.

The procedure applied to determine the sample size will be different for testing the hypothesis. The general method applied to derive the sample size is explained below.

Size of the Random Sample for Specified Precision

Chose a large sample from infinite large population.

Let $\bar{x}$ be the mean of large sample, and the mean of large population is equal to μ. The $\bar{x}$ is an unbiased estimate of the population.

Let E be the permissible error in estimation of population mean μ and confidence coefficient is $(1-\alpha)$, then we the investigator has to determine the sample size, which is written as n, such that

$$P\left[\left|\bar{x}-\mu\right|\leq E\right]=1-\alpha \qquad\qquad .....(8.1)$$

But for normal population or for large sample of any population, $\bar{x} \sim N\left(\mu, \sigma^2/n\right)$

When we chose 95% confidence coefficient, then

$$P\left[\left|\frac{\bar{x}-\mu}{\frac{\sigma}{\sqrt{n}}}\right|\leq 1.96\right]=0.95$$

$$.....(8.2)$$

Equate 1 and 2, then

$$E = 1.96\ \frac{\sigma}{\sqrt{n}}$$

$$\sqrt{n} = 1.96\ \frac{\sigma}{E}$$

Squaring both side

$$n = \frac{\left(1.96\right)^2 \sigma^2}{E^2} = \frac{\left(Z\alpha/2\right)^2 \sigma^2}{E^2}$$

Similarly we can obtain the sample size, when proportional values of sample and population are known is n= $\dfrac{PQ(Z\alpha/2)^2}{E^2}$

When P is not known , then n= $\dfrac{pq(Z\alpha/2)^2}{E^2}$, where p and q proportions of success and failure.

Example: In a clinical trial studies a random sample of 64 subjects were selected for study, the mean of B.P. was found to be 160 and variance is 100.

(i) Compute the 95% confidence limits for population mean

(ii) If the investigator wants in the 95% confidence, that the error in estimate of population mean should not exceed ± 1.4, how many additional number of patients are required?

Solution:

(a) Given that $n = 64$, $\bar{x}$ (Mean) $= 160$ and $s^2 = 100$

$$\therefore \qquad S = \sqrt{S^2} = \sqrt{100} = 10$$

Then the confidence limits are

$$\bar{x} \pm (1.96)\frac{S}{\sqrt{n}} = 160 \pm (1.96)\frac{10}{\sqrt{64}}$$

$=157.55 \text{-------} 162.45$

(b) To find n , given that $E = \pm 1.4$

$E^2 = (1.4)^2 = 1.96$

$$n = \frac{(Z\alpha/2)^2 S^2}{E^2}$$

$$n = \frac{(1.96)^2 10^2}{1.4^2} = 196$$

Hence the additional number of patients required $= 196 - 64 = 132$.

General Procedure for determining Sample Size

When we consider the population parameter as μ and sample value as $\bar{X}$ and δ is taken as difference between these two values, then $\delta = |\mu - \bar{X}|$. Let L be the half width of confidence interval, where $L = Z_{\alpha/2}$ SE($\bar{X}$),---------1

SE($\bar{X}$) is standard error of Mean and $Z_{\alpha/2}$ is Gaussian distribution value , which is selected on the basis of confidence level. Investigator can choose Z = 1.96 when $\alpha = 0.05$ and Z = 2.58 when $\alpha = 0.01$.

Since SE($\bar{X}$) included always the sample size N in the study and L will be specified, then the investigator can use the equation $L = Z_{\alpha/2}$ SE($\bar{X}$) to compute the sample size N.

When an investigator wishes to perform experiment on various subgroups, in that situation sample size should be computed separately for each subgroups.

When there are many parameters under consideration, then the investigator should look into to two main approaches to compute the sample size.

1. Compute the sample size for the most important parameters, when it is possible to identify.

2. Compute the sample size for all the parameters and select one of the largest values from that group. Latter it would give a better precision, than the expected one.

Example: If L = 1.5 and standard deviation of sample chosen for study is S= 6.4, then compute the sample size required for study.

Solution: Standard error is obtained by the equation $SE(\left(\overline{X}\right)) = \dfrac{S}{\sqrt{n}}$,

$$L = Z_{\alpha/2}SE\left(\overline{X}\right)$$

$$1.2 = 1.96 \times \dfrac{S}{\sqrt{n}} \ ,$$

$$1.2 = 1.96 \times \dfrac{6.4S}{\sqrt{n}} \ ,$$

Square both sides and cross multiplying the value we get $n = \dfrac{\left(1.96 \times 6.4\right)^2}{1.2^2}$

$$= 157.35/1.44$$
$$= 109.27$$
$$= 109$$

If the L is more precise one then, L = 0.4   then $n = \dfrac{\left(1.96 \times 6.4\right)^2}{0.4^2} = 983$, the sample size to be chosen for study is increased to 983 , when the value of L is enhanced or made it more smaller.

Mathematical Equation to estimate sample size in simple cases: These formulas are valid only for situations in which Gaussian approximation is applicable. Commonly used parameters in these situation are P and standard deviations σ . In case when P is not available, investigator can use P = 0.5. This will give maximum n. Similarly in case of sensitivity and specificity, which are considered as proportion, divide prevalence rate of disease for sensitivity and by (1 – prevalence) for specificity.

1. ***Sample size calculation when population proportion with specified absolute precision***: The mathematical equation used to calculate sample size is $n = \dfrac{pq(Z\alpha/_2)^2}{E^2}$ where p anticipated value of the proportion in the population, E is absolute precision required on either side of the proportion

   This is an equation which can be used for the determination of sample size during the II – Phase of clinical trials and survey.

Example 1: A group of 5 people took a project to make a survey to determine what proportion of families in a slum area medically indigent. In this project the investigator has put the condition that proportion should not be greater than 40%. The difference between the population and sample proportion d = 0.05. What should be the size of the family or sample to perform this project.?

Solution: Given that $Z_{\alpha/2}$ = 1.96, p = 0.40 and q = 0.60 and d = 0.05

$$\text{Then} \quad n = \frac{pq\left(Z_{\alpha/2}\right)^2}{E^2} = \frac{0.4 \times 0.6\left(1.96\right)^2}{0.05^2} = 368.79$$

Then the value will be rounded to the nearest value , n = 369.

Example 2: A study is conducted to compute the sample size when the current smoking rate of women in an organization is 25% and proportion difference is 2% (d =0.02). Compute the sample size needed for study.

$$n = \frac{pq\left(Z_{\alpha/2}\right)^2}{E^2} = \frac{0.25 \times 0.75\left(1.96\right)^2}{0.02^2} = 1801$$

1. **Sample size calculation when population mean with specified precision**

   The mathematical equation used to calculate sample size is n= $\dfrac{Z_\alpha^2 \sigma^2}{E^2}$ σ = The population standard deviation which can be obtained by a pilot study and E is absolute precision required on either side of mean.

   This method also can be used in II – Phase of clinical trial when the primary outcome is measured on a continuous scale, the focus is on mean. When $Z\alpha$ is considered as 1.96, then the equation can be written as n= $\dfrac{\left(1.96\right)^2 \sigma^2}{E^2}$, the $Z\alpha$ and E are arbitrarily and they are set by an investigator.

2. **Sample size calculation when difference between two population proportions with specified absolute precision and with equal in sample size.**

   The mathematical equation used to calculate sample size is

   $$\frac{Z_\alpha^2 / 2\left[P_{1(1-P_1)} + P_{2(1-P2)}\right]}{E^2}$$

   P_1 and P_2 are predicted or expected proportions in two populations and E is absolute precision required on either side of difference in proportion

3. **Sample size calculation when difference between means two population with specified absolute precision and with equal in sample size.**

   The mathematical equation used to calculate sample size is   n= $\dfrac{Z_\alpha^2\left(\sigma_1^2 + \sigma_2^2\right)}{E^2}$, σ_1 and σ_2 standard deviations of two population, they can be estimated from a pilot study and E is specified precision of the estimated difference on either side of the mean difference

4. Sample Size for testing for population proportion

$$n = \frac{\left[Z_\alpha^2/2\sqrt{P_{0(1-P_0)}} + Z\beta\sqrt{P_{1(1-P_1)}} \right]^2}{E^2}$$

where P_0 is the value of P under H_0, P_1 is the value of population proportion, which is medically very important. $\delta = (P_0 - P_1)$ is the difference which is to be detected

5. Sample size calculation for population mean with specified precision

The mathematical equation used to calculate sample size is $n = \dfrac{\sigma^2 \left(Z_{\alpha/2} + Z_\beta \right)^2}{\delta^2}$ σ = The population standard deviation, which can be estimated from pilot study. δ = The minimum difference between the means of H_0 and H_1

6. Sample Size calculation for difference between population proportions equal in size (n) of two groups

$$n = \frac{\left[Z_{a/2}\sqrt{P_{0(1-P_0)}} + Z\beta\sqrt{P_{1(1-P_1)}} \right]^2}{E^2}$$

P1 and P2 are the expected or anticipated proportions of two population and $\delta =(P_1 - P_2)$ is the difference P_1 and P_2 to be detected. $P = \dfrac{P_1 + P_2}{2}$

When null Hypothesis is considered then $H_0 : P_1 = P_2$

7. Sample Size calculation for difference between population means equal in size of two groups.

$$n = \frac{\left(\sigma_1^2 + \sigma_2^2 \right)\left(Z_{a/2} + Z_\beta \right)^2}{E^2}$$

, σ_1 and σ_2 standard deviations of two population, they can be estimated from a pilot study and they will equal in most of the cases and δ = The minimum difference between the means of under H_1 that is to be detected.

8. Sample Size calculation for independence in matched pairs.

$$n = \frac{\left[Z_{a/2}\sqrt{P_{10} + P_{01}} + Z\beta\sqrt{P_{10} + p_{01} - \left(P_{10} - p_{01}\right)^2} \right]^2}{\delta^2}$$

H0 : $P_{10} = P_{01}$ and P = ½

P_{10} and P_{01} are discordant probabilities, δ = difference between P_{10} and P_{01}

CHAPTER 9

Logistic Regression Analysis

Logistic Regression

We have studied regression analysis which involves only two variables as simple linear regression analysis. In general, the simple linear equation or model will be expressed in the form $Y = a + bx + \varepsilon$, where y is the arbitrary observed value of a continuous dependent variable and ε is the difference between observed value of Y and Predicted value Y. If ε is zero, then the regression equation can be written as $Y = a + bx$.

This simple regression model is not ideal when Y is taken as dichotomous or Binary variable, because the expected value of Y is the probability value, which is limited to range 0 through 1, It has been observed that the estimation of association between a primary exposure and a disease is usually less precise when it is necessary to stratify on many potential confounding variables simultaneously. The regression model is one way to achieve a link between different strata.

Here for designing a regression model, the investigator names the exposure variable as X in place of E, and the investigator will be interested to know the risk of D as it changes as the amount of exposure level is changed. The probability of exposure will be written as $P_x = P(D/X=x)$. Generally, investigator likes to draw the graph of P_x against x, that will explain everything about the risk of the disease, at all possible levels. This regression model provides the relationship between exposure and disease and also gives complete description.

Logistic regression is a statistical method for analyzing a dataset in which there are one or more than one independent variables to determine an outcome. The outcome is measured with a dichotomous variable (where there are only two possible outcomes).

Linear Model

The most common model which will be used in clinical research is linear model. The linear model can be written as $P_x = P(D/X = x) = a + bx$.

In this model, we assume that as the level of $X = x$ changes, the risk changes linearly. In this case the investigator considers the binary factors, they are named as 0 and 1.

If the subject is exposed to the risk factor X, then the binary number is considered as 1, if the subject is not exposed to the risk factor, then it is named as 0.

$$\begin{cases} \text{Exposed} = 1 \\ \text{Non - Exposed is} = 0 \end{cases}$$

For X = 0, we can obtain the parameter a, generally it is named as intercept. To obtain the next parameter b, investigator will consider two levels of exposure, that they differ by one unit on the scale X, say X = x + 1 and X = x. If X denotes the consumption of coffee per day, then the increase in consumption of coffee per day is written as X = x + 1

If P_x = a + bx then P_{x+1} = a + b(x + 1), the difference in the risk of disease D between x and x + 1 is written as

$$P_{x+1} - P_x = a + b(x + 1) - (a + bx)$$
$$= a + bx + b - a - bx$$
$$= b$$

The slope b is considered as excess risk, which is associated with a unit increase of x (Exposure) to x+1.

The excess risk associated with a unit increase in x does not depend on, which level of x the increase is measured from, but according to the linear assumption, the risk increases in a straight-line form.

Risk Factor		Disease Status		Total
		Death	No Death	
Exposed (x +1)		60	30	90
Non-Expose x		20	10	30
				120

Then $\qquad$ Px = 20/120 = 1/6 = 0.17

$\qquad$ Px + 1 = 60/120 = 1/2 = 0.5

$\qquad$ a = 0.17

$\qquad$ b = Px + 1 − Px = 0.5 − 0.17 = 0. 33

The linear equation is $\qquad$ Px = a + bx = 0.2 + 0.33x

The Log Linear Model

In clinical research the most often used method is to measure association between exposure and outcome event is log linear model, which is an alternative to the linear model.

This method measures the linearity in the relationship between the log risk and exposure level of the variables.

The log linear model will be written as

$$Log(Px) = log(P(D/X = x)) = a + bx$$

After taking the exponential both side, $e^{log(Px)} = e^{a+bx}$

$$P_{x} = P(D/X = x) = e^{a+bx}$$

The parameters may be interpreted as intercept and slope.

The value a is obtained as the log of risk, when the base line level X = 0, or P(D/X = 0) and it is given as e^a

Like linear model, when the exposure level is increased by one unit, then $\log(P_{x+1}) = \log(P(D/X = x +1)) = a + b(x + 1)$

Then $\log(P_{x+1}) - \log(P_x) = a + b(x + 1) - (a + bx) = b$

Then $\log\left(\dfrac{P_{(x+1)}}{P_x}\right) = b$

The value is considered as the relative risk due to increase in exposure by one unit.

Take the exponential both side, then $e^{\log\left(\frac{P_{(x+1)}}{P_x}\right)} = e^b$

$$\left(\dfrac{P_{(x+1)}}{P_x}\right) = e^b$$

Simple Linear Model

The important assumption made in this model is that the log odds of D changes linearly with changes in X.

The graph of logistic regression curves with the value of the risk, p, or with log odds, ie $\log(p/1-p)$ changes to line.

Here the shapes of the curves are resembling the probit model, but the coefficients a and b have some interpretation.

When $b = 0$ indicates there is no relationship between the risk of D and exposure X, , i.e., they are independent.

A positive value of b reflects increasing risk of D as exposure increases, and a negative value indicates decreasing risk as the level of exposure increases.

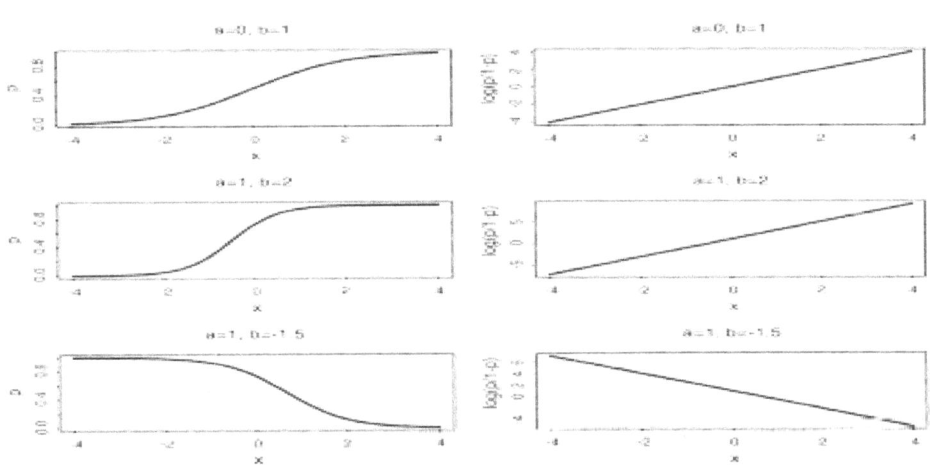

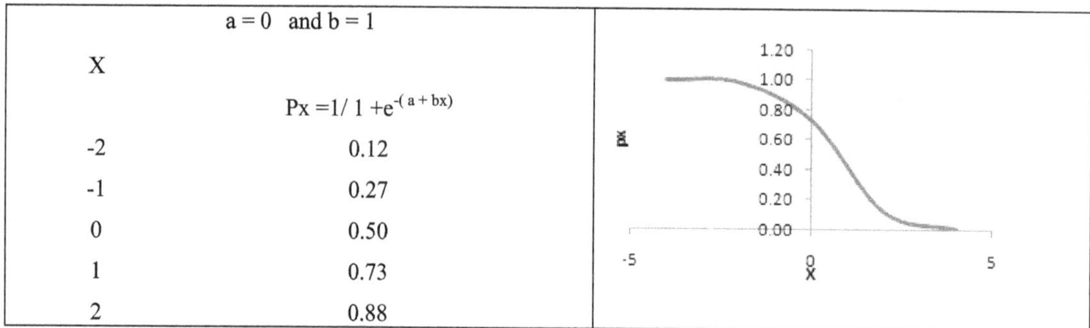

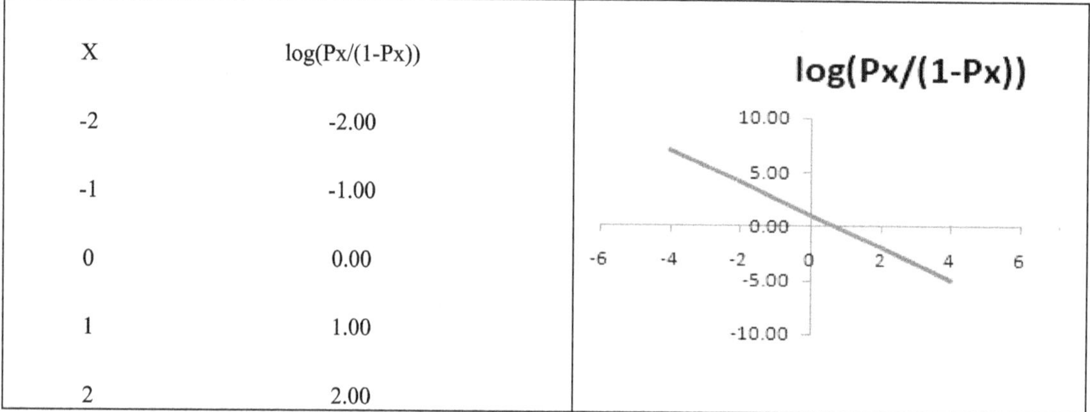

Example: From the following data, find that is there any association between inoculation and absence of attack of typhoid. Form the logistic regression and verify the level of significance using Chi-Square test.

	Attacked	Not Attacked
Inoculated	12	674
Not Inoculated	47	1122
Total	59	1796

Solution:

	Attacked	Not Attacked	Total
Inoculated	12	674	686
Not Inoculated	47	1122	1169
Total	59	1796	1855

$$P_0 = 12/686 = 0.0175$$
$$P_1 = 47/1169 = 0.0402$$
$$a = \ln(P_0) = \ln(0.0175) = -4.04597$$

$$\ln(P_1) = \ln(0.0402) = -3.21376$$
$$b = \ln(P_1) - \ln(P_0) = 0.832215$$
$$\text{Log}(P_x) = a + bx = -4.04597 + 0.832215.X$$

Probit Model

In probability theory and statistics, the **Probit** function is the quantile function associated with the standard normal distribution, which is commonly denoted as N(0,1). It has applications in exploratory statistical graphics and specialized regression modeling of binary response variables.

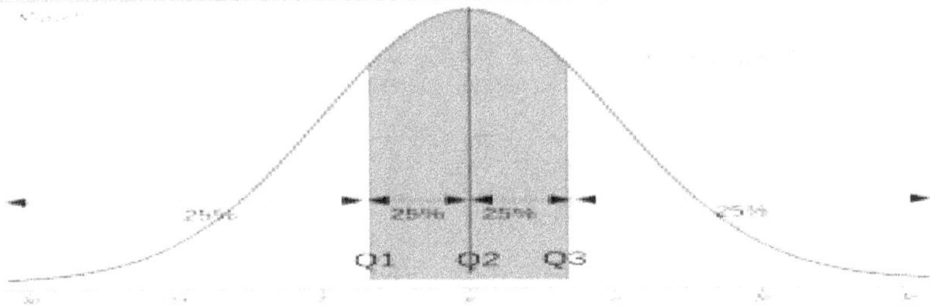

This model is designed to avoid the possibility of negative risks or the risk greater than 1 be choosing the relationship between x and Px , there the values cannot lie outside the range of 0 and 1

Generally the Probit model is given by the equation $Px = P(D/X = x) = ø(a + bx)$, here the value of a + bx is taken as u , then ø(u) is taken as the area under the standard normal distribution curve to the left of u. The value of u = a + bx always increases from very large negative to large positive and the area to the left of a+bx, increase from 0 to 1.

Probit model, is used to model dichotomous or binary outcome variables. In the probit model, the inverse standard normal distribution of the probability is modeled as a linear combination of the predictors.

For the Probit model P_0 is taken as ø(u), then a is obtained by using the standard Normal distribution table. If $P_0 = 0.0065 = ø(a)$, then a is obtained by comparing the corresponding ø(a) = 0.0065, that is area A = 0.0065 with Z value of the standard Normal distribution table then a = − 2.4847

If $P_1 = 0.0138$, then b= $(P_1-P_0) = (0.0138 - 0.0065) = 0.0073$

Then a + b = 0.0065 + 0.0073 = 0.0138, then ø(a +b) = ø(0.0138) = −2.2038

Then b = −2.2038 − a

= −2.2038 − (−2.4847)

= 0.2809

Then the Probit regression model can be written as Px = ø(−2.4847 + 0.2809x),

Number in the table represents P(Z ≤ z)

z	0.00	0.01	0.02	0.03	0.04	0.05	0.06	0.07	0.08	0.09
−3.6	.0002	.0002	.0001	.0001	.0001	.0001	.0001	.0001	.0001	.0001
−3.5	.0002	.0002	.0002	.0002	.0002	.0002	.0002	.0002	.0002	.0002
−3.4	.0003	.0003	.0003	.0003	.0003	.0003	.0003	.0003	.0003	.0002
−3.3	.0005	.0005	.0005	.0004	.0004	.0004	.0004	.0004	.0004	.0003
−3.2	.0007	.0007	.0006	.0006	.0006	.0006	.0006	.0005	.0005	.0005
−3.1	.0010	.0009	.0009	.0009	.0008	.0008	.0008	.0008	.0007	.0007
−3.0	.0013	.0013	.0013	.0012	.0012	.0011	.0011	.0011	.0010	.0010
−2.9	.0019	.0018	.0018	.0017	.0016	.0016	.0015	.0015	.0014	.0014
−2.8	.0026	.0025	.0024	.0023	.0023	.0022	.0021	.0021	.0020	.0019
−2.7	.0035	.0034	.0033	.0032	.0031	.0030	.0029	.0028	.0027	.0026
−2.6	.0047	.0045	.0044	.0043	.0041	.0040	.0039	.0038	.0037	.0036
−2.5	.0062	.0060	.0059	.0057	.0055	.0054	.0052	.0051	.0049	.0048
−2.4	.0082	.0080	.0078	.0075	.0073	.0071	.0069	.0068	.0066	.0064
−2.3	.0107	.0104	.0102	.0099	.0096	.0094	.0091	.0089	.0087	.0084
−2.2	.0139	.0136	.0132	.0129	.0125	.0122	.0119	.0116	.0113	.0110
−2.1	.0179	.0174	.0170	.0166	.0162	.0158	.0154	.0150	.0146	.0143
−2.0	.0228	.0222	.0217	.0212	.0207	.0202	.0197	.0192	.0188	.0183
−1.9	.0287	.0281	.0274	.0268	.0262	.0256	.0250	.0244	.0239	.0233
−1.8	.0359	.0351	.0344	.0336	.0329	.0322	.0314	.0307	.0301	.0294
−1.7	.0446	.0436	.0427	.0418	.0409	.0401	.0392	.0384	.0375	.0367
−1.6	.0548	.0537	.0526	.0516	.0505	.0495	.0485	.0475	.0465	.0455
−1.5	.0668	.0655	.0643	.0630	.0618	.0606	.0594	.0582	.0571	.0559
−1.4	.0808	.0793	.0778	.0764	.0749	.0735	.0721	.0708	.0694	.0681
−1.3	.0968	.0951	.0934	.0918	.0901	.0885	.0869	.0853	.0838	.0823
−1.2	.1151	.1131	.1112	.1093	.1075	.1056	.1038	.1020	.1003	.0985
−1.1	.1357	.1335	.1314	.1292	.1271	.1251	.1230	.1210	.1190	.1170
−1.0	.1587	.1562	.1539	.1515	.1492	.1469	.1446	.1423	.1401	.1379
−0.9	.1841	.1814	.1788	.1762	.1738	.1711	.1685	.1660	.1635	.1611
−0.8	.2119	.2090	.2061	.2033	.2005	.1977	.1949	.1922	.1894	.1867
−0.7	.2420	.2389	.2358	.2327	.2296	.2266	.2236	.2206	.2177	.2148
−0.6	.2743	.2709	.2676	.2643	.2611	.2578	.2546	.2514	.2483	.2451
−0.5	.3085	.3050	.3015	.2981	.2946	.2912	.2877	.2843	.2810	.2776
−0.4	.3446	.3409	.3372	.3336	.3300	.3264	.3228	.3192	.3156	.3121
−0.3	.3821	.3783	.3745	.3707	.3669	.3632	.3594	.3557	.3520	.3483
−0.2	.4207	.4168	.4129	.4090	.4052	.4013	.3974	.3936	.3897	.3859
−0.1	.4602	.4562	.4522	.4483	.4443	.4404	.4364	.4325	.4286	.4247
−0.0	.5000	.4960	.4920	.4880	.4840	.4801	.4761	.4721	.4681	.4641

Simple Logistic Regression

We have learned that $\log \dfrac{P_{(x)}}{1 - P_x} = \log(\text{ODDs of } D/X = x) = a + bx$

Take e both side of the equation, then $\dfrac{P_{(x)}}{1 - P_x} = e^{a + bx}$

Then $\dfrac{1}{e^{a+bx}} = \dfrac{1 - P_x}{P_x} = \dfrac{1}{P_x} - 1$

After taking 1 towards left hand side of the equation we get

$$\frac{1}{e^{a+bx}} + 1 = \frac{1}{P_x}$$

$$\frac{1 + e^{a+bx}}{e^{a+bx}} = \frac{1}{P_x}, \text{ then}$$

$$P_x = \frac{e^{a+bx}}{1 + e^{a+bx}}$$

or it can be written as $P_x = \dfrac{1}{1 + e^{-(a+bx)}}$

This is another way to express the relationship in terms of log odds associated with $P_{x\backslash}$

Example: If $Px = 1/\ 1 + e^{-(a+bx)}$

When $a = 0$ and $b = 1$

X	Px
−4	0.02
−2	0.12
0	0.50
1	0.73
2	0.88

The shape of the graph will be as shown below

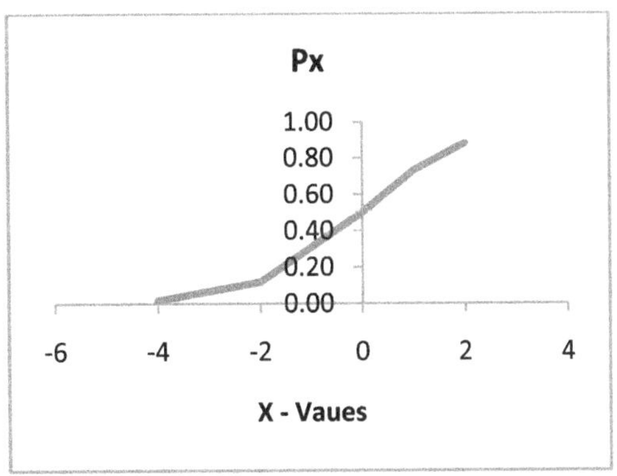

X	log(Px/1 − Px)
-4	-1.74
-2	-0.87
0	0.00
1	0.43
2	0.87

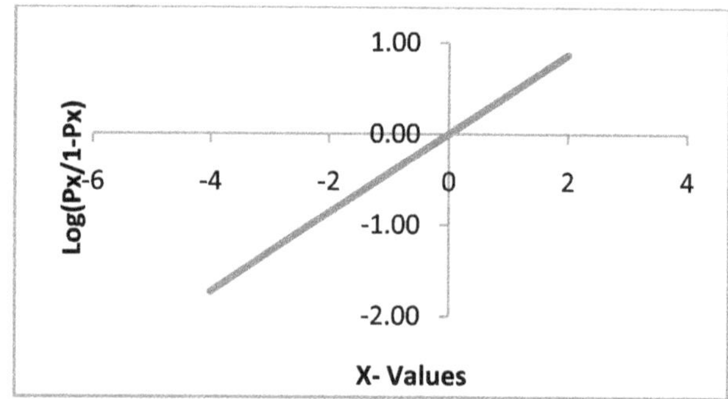

The logistic regression model deals with the case, where the random variable P_x of interest is a dichotomous variable taking the value 1 with probability P and 0 with the probability (1 –P).

Logistic regression analysis assumes that the relationship between Px and variate x.

Two important reasons that make the logistic regression model popular are

1. The range of logistic function is between 0 and 1.
2. The curve of logistic function has an increasing S-Shape, with a threshold, that makes more suitable for use as a Biological Model.

Slope of a Line Joining Two Points

Let A and B be the points (x_1, y_1) and (x_2, y_2) respectively. Let AB be inclined at an angle θ to the x-axis. Draw AL, BM $\perp$ to X-axis and AN $\perp$ to BM. OL = x_1, AL = y_1, OM = x_2, BM = y_2

Since AN is || to x-axis, $B\hat{A}N = \theta$

$$\text{The slope of AB} = \tan\theta = \frac{AN}{AB} = \frac{BM - NM}{LM} = \frac{BM - AL}{OM - OL} = \frac{y_2 - y_1}{x_2 - x_1}$$

$\therefore$ The slope of the line joining the two points (x_1, y_1) and (x_2, y_2) is $\dfrac{y_2 - y_1}{x_2 - x_1}$

For example, if $A \equiv (3, -4)$ and $B \equiv (-1, 5)$ the slope of AB $= \dfrac{y_2 - y_1}{x_2 - x_1} = \dfrac{5 - (-4)}{-1 - 3} = \dfrac{9}{-4} = -\dfrac{9}{4}$

Intercepts on x and y axes

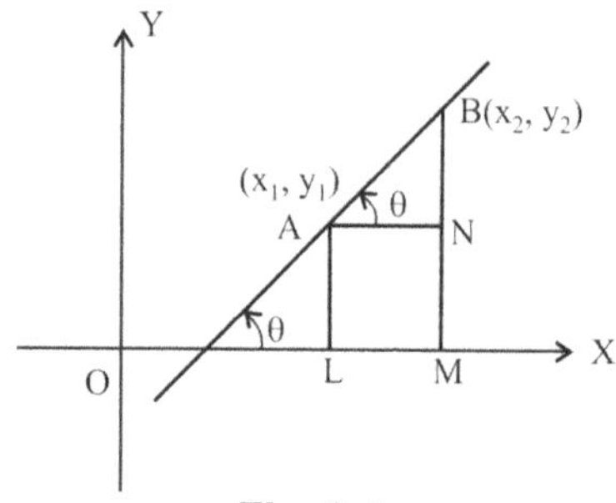

Fig. 9.1

Equation of a Straight Line Passing through Two Points

Let the straight line pass through the points A(x_1, y_1) an B(x_2, y_2). Let P(x, y) be any point on the line AB.

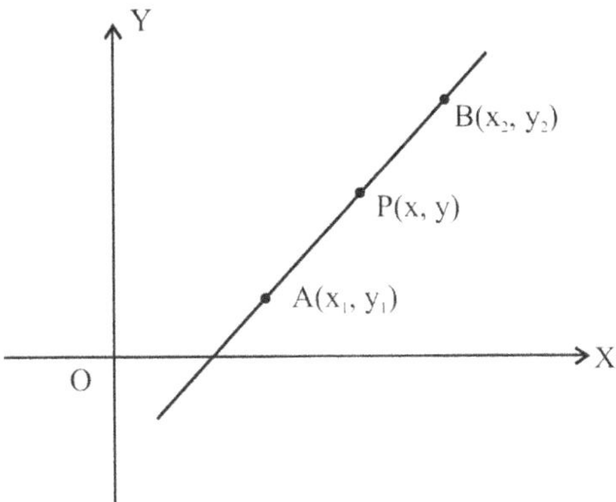

Fig. 9.2

Slope of $AP = \dfrac{y - y_1}{x - x_1}$; Slope of $AB = \dfrac{y_2 - y_1}{x_2 - x_1}$

Since A, P, B lie on the same line, slope of AP = slope of AB

i.e., $\qquad \dfrac{y - y_1}{x - x_1} = \dfrac{y_2 - y_1}{x_2 - x_1}$

Hence the equation of the line passing through the points (x_1, y_1) and (x_2, y_2) is

$$\dfrac{y - y_1}{x - x_1} = \dfrac{y_2 - y_1}{x_2 - x_1}$$

$$(y - y_1) = \left(\dfrac{y_2 - y_1}{x_2 - x_1} \right)(x - x_1)$$

Same procedure can be applied to form linear equation and logistic regression equation when binary exposures X=0 and X= 1 are considered in epidemiological study.

Example 1:

Risk Factor	Disease Status		
	Death	No Death	Total
Exposed (x +1)	60	30	90
Non-Expose x	20	50	70
	80	40	120

Then $Px = 20/70 = 2/7 = 0.29$

$Px + 1 = 60/90 = 2/3 = 0.67$

$a = 0.29$

$b = Px + 1 - Px = 0.67 - 0.29 = 0.38$

The linear equation is $Px = a + bx = 0.29 + 0.38x$

When we consider the log Linear model

$a = \log(P_0) = \ln(0.29) = -1.25$

$b = \log(P_1/P_0) = \log(0.67/0.29) = 0.85$

$\text{Log}(Px) = -1.25 + 0.85x$

***Example* 2:** Data recorded about an incidence study is summarized in the following table. Form the logistic regression model.

Risk Factor ↓	Disease Status		
	Disease	No Disease	Total
Exposed	10	08	18
Non-Exposed	3	979	982
	13	987	1000

Solution:

Then $Px = 03/982 = 0.003$

$Px+1 = 10/18 = 2/3 = 0.67 = 0.556$

$a = 0.003$

$b = Px+1 - Px = 0.556 - 0.003 = 0.553$

The linear equation is $Px = a + bx = 0.003 + 0.553x$

When we consider the log Linear model

$a = \text{Log}(P_0) = \ln(0.003) = -5.791$

$b = \log(P_1/P_0) = \log(0.0.553/0.003) = 5.203$

$\text{Log}(Px) = -5.791 + 5.203x$

The value of b can be obtained by using the formula to find slope between two points (x_1, y_1)

and (x_2, y_2) $m = \dfrac{y_2 - y_1}{x_2 - x_1}$

In this problem $(x_1, y_1) = (0, 0.003)$ and $(x_2, y_2) = (1, 0.556)$

Slope $b = \dfrac{y_2 - y_1}{x_2 - x_1} = \dfrac{0.556 - 0.003}{1 - 0} = 0.553$

$$(y - y_1) = \left(\dfrac{y_2 - y_1}{x_2 - x_1}\right)(x - x_1)$$

$$(Y - 0.003) = \frac{0.556 - 0.003}{1 - 0}(X - 0)$$

$$Y - 0.003 = 0.553X$$

$$Px - 0.003 = 0.553X$$

$$Px = 0.003 + 0.553X, \text{ Y is replaced by Px}$$

Then the linear equation can be written as $Px = a + bx = 0.003 + 0.553x$

Or

$$\text{Take } \ln(a) = \ln(0.003) = -5.791 \text{ and } \left(\frac{y_2 - y_1}{x_2 - x_1}\right) = \ln\left(\frac{0.556 - 0.003}{1 - 0}\right) = \ln(0.553) = 5.203$$

$$\log(Px) = -5.791 + 5.203x$$

***Example* 3**: A group employees in health profession were given questionnaire and they were asked one question, whether they currently smoke or not. The vital status of these employees was ascertained by an investigator after two years (follow-up) of study period. The data tabulated in the table enumerates those who died due to CVD after two years due to smoking. Form he logistic regression equation and also 95% confidence interval.

Smokers	Disease Status		Total
	Disease	No Disease	
Yes (Exposed)	30	1390	1417
No-(Non-Exposed)	16	1879	1898
	46	3269	3315

Solution:

$$P(D/E) \qquad P1 = 30/1417 = 0.021$$

$$P(D/NE) \qquad P0 = 16 / 1898 = 0.008$$

$$a = P_0 = 0.008$$

$$b = P_1 - P_0 = 0.013$$

$$OR = P_1/P_0 = 2.625$$

$$SE = \sqrt{\frac{1}{a} + \frac{1}{b} + \frac{1}{c} + \frac{1}{d}}$$

$$SE = \sqrt{\frac{1}{31} + \frac{1}{1390} + \frac{1}{16} + \frac{1}{1879}} = 0.3116$$

95% Confidence interval is CI

$$L_{\log} = \ln(OR) + 1.96 \times SE = 0.35434$$

$$= \ln(2.625) + 1.96 \times SE$$

$$= 0.35434$$

$$U_{log} = \ln(OR) - 1.96 \times SE$$

$$= \ln(2.625) + 1.96 \times SE$$

$$= 1.57582$$

$$L = e(L_{log}) = 1.4252$$

$$U = \exp(U_{log}) = 4.8347$$

$$a = -4.8283$$

$$b = 0.4855$$

$$\log(Px) = -4..8283 + 0.4855x$$

***Example* 4:** The data given below is about relationship between gestational age of infant is X (In the form weeks) at the time of birth and whether the infant was breast feeding at the time of discharge from the hospital (not feeding is coded as 0 and feeding is coded as 1). Compute odd ratio and logs of odds for the data listed in the table.

X-Age (In terms Week)	Milk feeding status Y	
	YES -1	NO -0
24-X-0	2	4
25-X-1	2	3
26-X-2	7	2
27-X-3	7	2
28-X-4	16	4
29-X-4	14	1

Compute Probability of Y, Odds ratio of Y and Log of ODDS for each value of X

Solution: The observed probability of Y when Y=1 calculated as the ratio of the number of instances to the total number of instances of Y for that level

$$Py = P(D/X = x) = \text{Number of cases / Total number at a particular gestational age}$$

X-Age (In terms Week)	Milk feeding status Y		
	YES -1	NO -0	Total
24-X-0	2	4	6
25-X-1	2	3	5
26-X-2	7	2	9
27-X-3	7	2	9
28-X-4	16	4	10
29-X-4	14	1	15

(a) For Age X = 24, Py = (2/6) = 0.3333, ODDs = (Py/(1 – Py)) = (0.3333/(1-0.3333)) = 0.4999, Log(ODD) = ln(0.4999) = –0.6933

(b) For Age X = 25, Py = (2/5) = 0.4000 = ODDs = (Py/(1 – Py)) =(0.4000/(1 – 0.4000)) = 0.6667, Log(ODDS) = Ln(0.6667) = –0.4055

(c) For Age X = 26, Py = (7/9) = 0.7778 = ODDs = (Py/(1 – Py)) =(0.7778/(1 – 0.7778)) = 3.5000, Log(ODDS) = Ln(3.5000) = 1.2528

(d) For Age X = 27, Py = (7/9) = 0.7778 = ODDs = (Py/(1 – Py)) = (0.7778/(1 – 0.7778)) = 3.5000, Log(ODDS)=Ln(3.5000) = 1.2528

(e) For Age X = 28, Py = (16/20) = 0.8000 = ODDs = (Py/(1 – Py)) = (0.8000/(1 – 0.8000)) = 4.0000, Log(ODDS) = Ln(4.0000) = 1.3863

(f) For Age X = 29, Py = (14/15) = 0.9333 = ODDs = (Py/(1 – Py)) = (0.9333/(1 – 0.9333)) = 14.0000, Log(ODDS) = Ln(14.0000) = 2.6391

Advantages of the Logistic

1. Allows properties of a linear regression model to be exploited
2. The logit itself can take values between $-\infty$ and $+\infty$
3. Probability remains constrained between 0 and 1
4. The logit can be directly related to odds of disease

$$\ln\left(\frac{P}{1-P}\right) = \alpha + \beta x$$

$$\frac{P}{1-P} = e^{\alpha+\beta x}$$

Interpretation of coefficient β

The probabilities for an individual to fall into categories of exposure to a risk factor and presence or absence of disease are defined below:

	Exposure (E)	
Disease (D)	**YES**	**NO**
Yes	$P(y\|x = 1)$	$P(y\|x = 0)$
NO	$1-P(y\|x = 1)$	$1-P(y\|x = 0)$

$$\left(\frac{P}{1-P}\right) = e^{\alpha+\beta x}$$

$$\text{Odds}(D|E) = e^{\alpha+\beta}$$

$$\text{Odds}(D/\overline{E}) = e^{\alpha}$$

$$\text{OR} = \frac{e^{\alpha+\beta}}{e^{\alpha}}$$

$$\ln(\text{OR}) = \beta$$

Difference between probit and logistic regression

Probit	Logistic
The Probit model is link a function	A logistic regression uses a logit link function
And a probit regression uses an inverse normal link function: $$f(\mu_y) = \phi^{-1}(P)$$	A logistic regression uses a logit link function $$f(\mu_y) = \ln\left(\frac{P}{1-P}\right)$$
Coefficients for probit models can be interpreted as the difference in Z score associated with each one-unitdifference in the predictor variable.	Coefficient of logit $b = \log(P_{x+1}) - \log(P_x)$ $$= a + b(x+1) - (a+bx)$$ $$= b$$
The range of Probit function is between $-\infty$ to $+\infty$	The range of logistic function is between 0 and 1.
The relationship between probability and the predictors isn't linear	The relationship between probability and the predictors is linear

Difference between Linear Regression Model and Logistic Regression Model

Linear regression model	Logistic regression model
Linear Regression is a supervised regression model	Logistic Regression is a supervised classification model.
Here no activation function is used.	Here activation function is used to convert a linear regression equation to the logistic regression equation like ln(natural log)
Here no threshold value is needed.	Here a threshold value is added.
Here we calculate Root Mean Square Error(RMSE) to predict the next weight value.	Here we use precision to predict the next weight value.
Here dependent variable should be numeric, and the response variable is continuous to value.	Here the dependent variable consists of only two categories. Logistic regression estimates the odds outcome of the dependent variable given a set of quantitative or categorical independent variables.
It is based on the least square estimation.	It is based on maximum likelihood estimation.
Here when we plot the training datasets, a straight line can be drawn that touches maximum plots.	Any change in the coefficient leads to a change in both the direction and the steepness of the logistic function. It means positive slopes result in an S-shaped curve and negative slopes result in a Z-shaped curve.
Linear regression assumes the normal or Gaussian distribution of the dependent variable.	Logistic regression assumes the binomial distribution of the dependent variable

Measures of Association

The Main objective for using logistic model to measure the strength or a statistical relationship between the binary dependent variable and independent variable or covariant measurement , which are obtained from patients. This may help us to take important decision in patient management. In epidemiological study, logistic model uses odd ratio for measuring association.

The logistic regression model of P_X for X=0 and X=1 is written as

$$Log(OR) = log\left[\frac{Odd\ of\ D\ /\ X = 1}{Odd\ of\ D\ /\ X = 0}\right]$$

Here the odds of D/X = 1 is $P_1/1\text{-}P_1$ and odds for D/X=0 is $P_0/1 - P_0$

$$\text{Then } log(OR) = log\left[\frac{P_1\ /1 - P_1}{P_0\ /1 - P_0}\right] = log(P_1/1 - P_1) - log(P_0/1 - P_0)$$

$$= a + b \times 1 - a - b \times 0$$

$$= a + b - a - 0 = b$$

Then the parameter a is considered as log(OR) for X = 0 , here a = $log(P_0/1\text{-}P_0)$

If X has more discrete (Numerical) level , say X = x + 1 and X= x the

$$Log(OR) = log\left[\frac{Odd\ of\ D\ /\ X = x + 1}{Odd\ of\ D\ /\ X = x}\right]$$

$$= log\left[\frac{P_{x+1}\ /1 - P_{x+1}}{P_{x/1 - Px}}\right] = log(P_x + _1/1 - P_{x+1}) - log(P_x/1 - P_x)$$

$$= a + b(x + 1) - a - bx$$

$$= a + bx + b - a - bx$$

$$= b$$

So after taking exponential both side OR = e^b

Then the confidence interval can be obtained by using the equation $e^{[b\pm1.96\ SE(OR)]}$ for 95% confidence interval

$$\text{Where SE} = \sqrt{\frac{1}{a} + \frac{1}{b} + \frac{1}{c} + \frac{1}{d}}$$

Similarly for 99% confidence interval is $e^{[b\pm2.58\ SE(OR)]}$

Application of Logistic Regression

Logistic regression is a statistical method for predicting binary classes. The outcome or target variable is binary in nature.

For example, it can be used for cancer detection problems.

Logistic Regression predicts the probability of occurrence of a binary event utilizing a logit function. Logistic regression uses maximum likelihood estimation (MLE) to obtain the model coefficients that relate predictors to the target and also log(p/1-p) is the link function. Logarithmic transformation on the outcome variable allows us to model a non-linear association in a linear way. This is the equation used in Logistic Regression

The use of logistic regression analysis is widely applicable to epidemiologic studies concerned with quantifying an association between a study factor (i.e., an exposure variable) and a health outcome (i.e., disease status).

Techniques for both unconditional and conditional maximum likelihood estimation of the parameters in the logistic model are described and illustrated.

A general analysis strategy is also presented which incorporates the assessment of both interaction and confounding in quantifying an exposure-disease association of interest.

Logistic regression is used in various fields, most often in medical fields to analyze the data of epidemiological studies.

For example, the Trauma and Injury Severity Score (TRISS), w1ich is widely used to predict mortality in injured patients, was originally developed by Boyd *et al.* using logistic regression.

Many other medical scales used to assess severity of a patient have been developed using logistic regression.

Logistic regression may be used to predict the risk of developing a given disease (e.g. diabetes, Coronary heart disease) on observed characteristics of the patient (age, sex, body mass index, results of various blood tests etc.).

Interpretation of Logistic Regression Parameters

We turn into the interpretation of the two parameters, the intercept and the slope b of the logistic regression model, 1 and 2

$$Px = P(D/X = x) = a + bx \qquad .....(9.1)$$

$$Log(Px) = Log(P(D/X = x) = a + bx \qquad .....(9.2)$$

Here the exposure variable is taken as X and that takes on only two values, say, X=1 (exposed) and X=0 (unexposed).

Here the investigator will understand the meaning of a and b after analyzing the complete derivation.

When an investigator consider X=0, then the value of $log(P_0/1-P_0)=a+(b \times 0)=a$. It explains that a is obtained by taking log odds of disease D due to the unexposed variable.

In addition, comparing the exposed to the unexposed yields the Odds Ratio,

$$Log(OR) = log\left(\frac{Odds\ of\ D\ /\ X = 1}{Odds\ of\ D\ /\ X = 0}\right)$$

$$\text{Log(OR)} = \log\left(\frac{p_1/(1-p_1)}{p_0/(p_0-1)}\right)$$

$$\text{Log(OR)} = \log[p_1/(1-p_1)] - \log[(p_0/(1-p_0)]$$
$$= a + b \times 1 - (a + b \times 0)$$
$$= b$$

Thus, the slope parameter b is can be considered as the log Odds Ratio.

If X has several discrete (numerical) levels or is measured on a continuous scale, there is no change in the interpretation of a (the log odds of D when $X=0$).

To understand the concept of slope parameter $b,$ here we have to consider two exposure levels with a difference by one unit on the scale of $X,$

say, $X=x+1$ and $X=x.$ Then the log Odds Ratio comparing these two exposure groups is

$$\text{Log(OR)} = \log\left(\frac{\text{Odds of } D/X=1}{\text{Odds of } D/X=x}\right)$$

$$\text{Log(OR)} = \log\left(\frac{px+1/(1-px+1)}{px/(px-1)}\right)$$

$$\text{Log(OR)} = \log[px+1/(1-px+1)] - \log[(px/(1-px)]$$
$$= a + b\times(x+1) - (a + b\times x)$$
$$= b$$

Thus, b is the log Odds Ratio which is obtained by two exposure groups when their exposure increased by 1 unit on the unit scale $X.$ that will measure the log Odds Ratio which is associated between X and X+1.

But that Odds Ratio, associated with a unit increase in $X,$ does not depend on the choice of the baseline value X from which this unit increase is measured.

For example, if X measures coffee consumption in cups/day, the model Equation 2 indicates that the log Odds Ratio comparing exposures of 2 and 1 cigar /day is $b,$ this can be applied for 3 or 4 or 5 cups coffee or cigar per day.

Both of these comparisons correspond to the increase in exposure variable X by of 1 unit on the scale which is selected by the investigator.

Hence the value of b is therefore intimately connected to the particular exposure scale used.

Different (albeit closely related) slope parameters would be needed if you measure the risk factor age (X) in years as against months; in the first case, a unit increase in X corresponds to a 1 year age difference, whereas with the second choice it corresponds to only a 1 month age difference.

Since the term $e^{(a+bx)}$ is always positive, then the value of p_x must lie between 0 and 1 for any choice of the parameters a and b and at any level of the exposure $X.$

Here one can easily estimate the logistic regression slope parameter from data obtained from any design like case-control study and cohort study also.

Multiple Logistic Regression Model

Investigator often are much interested in establishing the relationships between several independent variables to measure one of the response or dependent or outcome variable. In this model these independent variables are risk factors which are labeled as X_1, X_2,-----X_k. These risk factors or variables may be either continuous or discrete or the combination of both. At given exposure levels, say $X_1 = x_1$, $X_2 = x_2$, ----------$X_0 = x_k$, then the investigator use P_{x1}, P_{x2},------P_{xk} to denote $P(D/X_1 = x_1, X_2 = x_2,----X_k = x_k)$

Then the Multiplicative logistic regression model can constructed as

$$\text{Log}\left(\frac{P_{x_1 x_2 ....x_k}}{1 - P_{x_1 x_2 x_3 ....x_k}}\right) = \log(P(D/X_1 = x_1, X_2 = x_2 -----X_k = x_k) = a + bx$$

$$= a + b_1 x_1 + b_2 x_2 + ---------- + b_k x_k$$

After taking exponential both side of the equation and after simplifying in the same way as simple logistic regression equation, we obtain

$$P_{x_1 x_2 ....x_k} = \frac{1}{1 + e^{-(a + b_1 x_1 + b_2 x_2 + ...+ b_k x_k)}}$$

To verify the risk of D changes, holding remaining risk factors x_2, x_3,-----x_k as fixed. In case of simple logistic model, the parameter a is obtained by obtaining the value of $\log(P_0 / 1 - P_0)$, here also we can obtain by computing $\log(P_{0,0---0}/(1 - P_{0,0---0})) = a$.

So that a can be considered as the log(ODDs of D) at the baseline level , where all the risk variables or factors are zero on their respective scales.

To obtain the slopes parameters b_1, b_2,----b_k, consider the comparison of two groups, whose risk factor or variable X_1 increase by 1 unit on the scale of X_1 and the remaining risk factors share the identical value.

If $X_1 = x_{1+1}$, $X_2 = x_2$ ---- $X_k = x_k$ then the difference in log(odds) of D of these two groups is

$$[a + b_1 x_1 + b_2 x_2 + ----------+b_k z_k] - [a + b_1 x_1 + b_2 x_2 + ----------+b_k x_k] = b1$$

Similarly the parameters b_2, b_3,----b_k can be obtained with a unit increase in the respective scale xj for j = 2,3,4----k.

Here the log(ODDs) ratio does not depend on the value of xj from which one unit increase has been considered and also odds ratio which is associated with changes in xj, is not affected by the values, which are considered as fixed in the model.

In case of multiple regression model, investigator assumes that, there is no interaction between xj and the other variables. This model is still linear, because the independent variables appear only in the first order, this feature is rather difficult to check, because we don't have scatter diagram to rely on as incase of simple linear regression.

Logistic Regression with Case-control Data

When we design a case-control for the population under study, when we assume how regression model can explain the risk of disease D depends on exposure variable X. Here we consider one outcome variable D and Exposure variable X, the logistic regression assumption gives $\log(Px/1-Px) = a + bx$, where $Px = P(D/X = x)$.

If π_{case} is the probability of an individual being sampled when they are in case or having disease, that can be written as P(Sampled/D).

When the control group is considered then the $\pi_{control} = P(\text{Sampled} / \bar{D})$. In this case probabilities or sampling fractions are not depending on the exposure level X. Here we can divide subpopulation which are exposed to exposure level $X = x$ into four part , on the basis of their disease status and whether they are included in the sample or not. Here the investigator can also measure relative frequency of these group from the subpopulation chosen for case-control study.

The Probability of case and sample with an exposure group $X = x$, then P(D & sampled /X=x) $= P(D/X = x)P(\text{Sampled}/D, X = x) = \pi_{case}P_x$

The four parts or groups with their respective proportions within the subpopulation with exposure $X = x$ are

1. Individual in a case and sampled : Proportion $= \pi_{case}P_x$

2. Individual in a case and sampled : Proportion $= (1 - \pi_{case})P_x$

3. Individual in a control and sampled : Proportion $= \pi_{control}(1 - P_x)$

4. Individual in a control and sampled : Proportion $= (1 - \pi_{control})((1 - P_x)$

The P(D|X = x, sampled) $= \left(\dfrac{\pi_{case}P_x}{\pi_{case}\,P_x + \pi_{control}\left(1 - P_x\right)} \right)$, this is based 1 & 3 group.

When the equation $\log(Px/1 - Px) = a + bx$, where $Px = P(D/X = x)$, then the

$$\log(Px/1 - Px) = \log\left(\frac{\pi_{case}P_x}{\pi_{control}\left(1 - P_x\right)} \right)$$

$$= \log\left(\frac{\pi_{case}}{\pi_{control}} \right) + \log\left(\frac{P_x}{\left(1 - P_x\right)} \right)$$

$$= \log\left(\frac{\pi_{case}}{\pi_{control}} \right) + a + bx$$

$$= a_1 + a + bx$$

$$= a^* + bx$$

$$a^* = \log\left(\frac{\pi_{case}}{\pi_{control}} \right) + a$$

Effect Modification

Consider the multiple logistic regression model $P_x = \dfrac{1}{1 + e^{-(a + b_1 x_1 + b_2 x_2 + b_3 x_3)}}$

The Parameter b_1 and b_2 are not same, because of the cross product value $b_3 = x_1 x_2$

Here the investigator assumes that both risk factor X_1 and X_2 are binary.

Example: Construct the multiple logistic regression models for the data listed in the following table

	HEART ATTACK	
BODY WEIGHT	**YES**	**NO**
≤150	30	540
150+-160	26	500
160+-170	45	580
170+-180	60	490
>180	75	730
Total	236	2840

Solution:

	HEART ATTACK		
BODY WEIGHT	**YES**	**NO**	**Total**
≤150	30	540	570
150+-160	26	500	526
160+-170	45	580	625
170+-180	60	490	550
>180	75	730	805
Total	236	2840	3076

MODEL 1

P	236/3076	0.0767
a	$\ln(P/(1-P))$	−2.487

Model2		**Diseases Status (Heart Attack)**		
		YES	**NO**	
Behaviour Type X	A -1	168	1400	1568
	B -0	68	1440	1508
		236	2840	3076

MODEL 3

HEART ATTACK

BODY WEIGHT	YES	NO	Total
≤150	30	540	570
150+-160	26	500	526
160+-170	45	580	625
170+-180	60	490	550
>180	75	730	805
Total	236	2840	3076

P0	30/570	0.0526
a	$\ln(P0/(1 - P_0))$	−2.8904
P1	26/526	0.058
	$\ln(P_1/(1 - P_1))$	−2.9565
$b_1 =$	$\ln(P_1/(1 - P_1)) - \ln(P_0/(1 - P_0))$	−0.0661

Using slope between two points, here points

(0, Ln(P$_0$/(1-P$_0$))= (0, -2.8904) and
(1, Ln(P$_1$/(1-P$_1$)) = (1, −2.9565)

$$b_1 = \frac{y_2 - x_1}{x_2 - x_1} = \frac{-0.9565 - (-2.8904)}{1 - 0}$$

$$= -0.0661 \qquad\qquad -0.0661$$

P_2	45/625	0.072
	$\ln(P_2/(1 - P_2))$	−2.5564
b_2	$\ln(P_2/(1 - P_2)) - \ln(P0/(1 - P0))$	0.334

Using slope between two points
(0, ln(P$_0$/(1-P$_0$)= (0, −2.8904) and (1,
Ln(P$_2$/(1-P$_2$))= (1, −2.5564)

$$b_2 = \frac{y_2 - x_1}{x_2 - x_1} = \frac{-2.5564 - (-2.8904)}{1 - 0} \qquad 0.334$$

$$= 0.334/1 = 0.334$$

P_3	60/550	0.1091
	$\ln(P_3/(1 - P_3)$	−2.1000
b_3	$\ln(P_3/(1 - P_3) - \ln(P_0/(1 - P_0))$	0.790

Using slope between two points
(0, ln(P0/(1 − P0) = (0, −2.8904) and (1,
Ln(P2/(1 − P2))= (1, −2.1000)

$$b_3 = \frac{y_2 - y_1}{x_2 - x_1} = \frac{-2.1000 - (-2.8904)}{1 - 0}$$

$$= 0.790/1 = 0.790$$

$$0.790$$

P_4	75/805	0.095
	$\ln(P_4/(1 - P_4))$	−2.2756
b_4	$\ln(P_4/(1 - P_4)) - \ln(P_0/(1 - P_0))$	0.615

Using slope between two points
(0, ln(P0/(1-P0)= (0, −2.8904) and
(1, Ln(P2/(1 − P2))= (1, −2.2756)

$$b_4 = \frac{y_2 - y_1}{x_2 - x_1} = \frac{-2.2759 - (-2.8904)}{1 - 0}$$

$$= 0.615/1 = 0.615$$

$$0.615$$

The Multiple logistic regression model is $Log(Px/1 - Px) = a + b_1x_1 + b_2x_2 + b_3x_3 + b_4x_4$
$$= -2.8904 - 0.0661 \times x_1 + 0.334 \times x_2 + 0.790 \times x_3 + 0.615 \times x_4$$

Logistic Regression Model Parameters

Here the investigator focus about the estimation of the parameters of a particular population model using the data chosen randomly from a sample.

Example: The data given below about the CHD event (outcome event) and body weight (Independent variable) of different category gives the detail about case group (no of subjects who got Disease) and the control group (number of subjects who did not get the disease). Compute Intercept and slopes for different category of body weight for the corresponding case and control group and fit the logistic regression model.

CHD Event

		Case - Disease (D)	Control NO Disease	Total
	≤ 140	30 a_1	550 b_1	$c_1 = 580$
Body	$x_1 = 140\text{-}150$	35 a_2	500 b_2	$c_2 = 535$
Weight (lb)	$x_2 = 150\text{-}160$	60 a_3	600 b_3	$c_3 = 660$
	$x_3 = 160\text{-}170$	70 a_4	510 b_4	$c_4 = 580$
	$x_4 => 170$	90 a_5	750 b_5	$c_5 = 840$
	Total	285	2910	3195

	Equation to Compute probability value of an event	Probability	Equation to obtain Intercept and Slopes	Intercept and Slopes
Computation of Intercept and Slopes	$\ln((a_1/c_1)/(b_1/c_1))$	$-2.91 = P_0$	$a = P_0$	-2.91
	$\ln((a_2/c_2)/(b_2/c_2))$	$-2.66 = P_1$	$b_1 = P_1 - P_0$	0.25
	$\ln((a_3/c_3)/(b_3/c_3))$	$-2.30 = P_2$	$b_2 = P_2 - P_0$	0.61
	$\ln((a_4/c_4)/(b_4/c_4))$	$-1.99 = P_3$	$b_3 = P_3 - P_0$	0.92
	$\ln((a_5/c_5)/(b_5/c_5))$	$-2.12 = P_4$	$b_4 = P_4 - P_0$	0.79

The Multiple logistic regression model is $Log(Px/1 - Px) = a + b_1x_1 + b_2x_2 + b_3x_3 + b_4x_4$
$$= -2.91 + 0,25 \times x_1 + 0.61 \times x_2 + 0.92 \times x_3 + 0.79 \times x_4$$

Likelihood Function

Before going for the Logistic regression model, we introduce the concept of Likelihood function. Generally, the likelihood function expresses the plausibility the quality of seeming reasonable or probable of different parameters values for a given data which is collected from a sample.

The likelihood function describes a hyper surface who's peak if it exits, represents the combination of model parameter values that the probability of drawing the sample obtained.

The likelihood function is usually defined differently for discrete and continuous probability distribution. The idea of likeliness is subjective. We can formally quantify such a concept through the use of likelihood function P, it is defined as L = P(data/p) , it is a conditional Probability and the L value of data(x) depends on p.

This likelihood function can be verified by considering the Binomial distribution, Poisson distribution and normal distribution.

1. For a Binomial distribution $L(X, P) = {}^{N}C_X \, P^X \, P^{(N-X)}$, that leads to $\hat{P} = \dfrac{X}{N}$

2. For a Poisson Distribution $L(X, \lambda) = \pi_{i=1}^{N} \, \dfrac{1^X e^{-1}}{x!}$, that leads to $\hat{\lambda} = \dfrac{\Sigma x_i}{n}$

Example: When hundred patients were suffering due to asthma were administered a new drug. 35 patients recovered and 65 have been not recovered from the disease. Find likelihood function of the probability of recovery for different values of P and Plot the graph of Likelihood and Log likelihood against P and also verify for what value of P L is maximum.

N	X	N-X	FACT(N)	FACTP(N-X)	FACT(X)	FACT
100	35	65	9.3326E+157	8.24765E+90	1.03331E+40	1.09507E+27

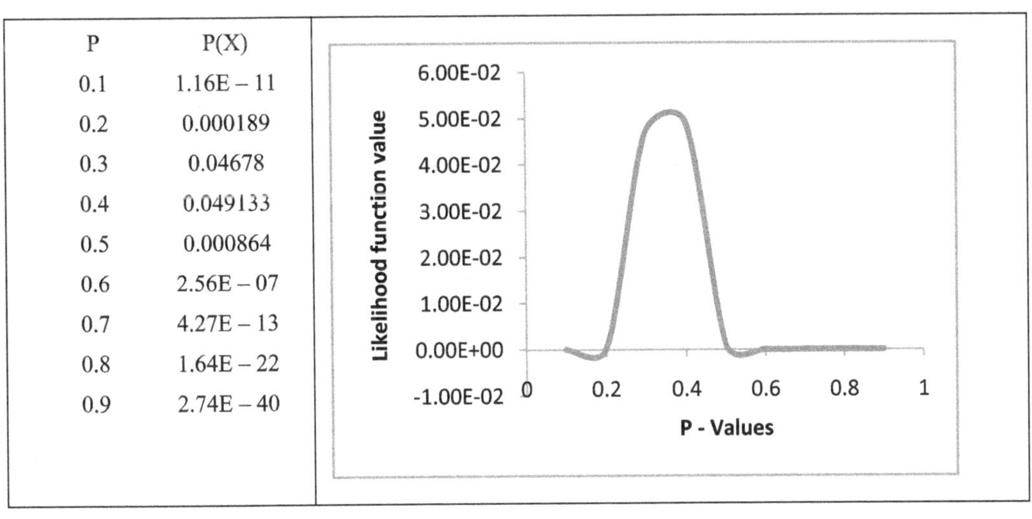

P	P(X)
0.1	$1.16E-11$
0.2	0.000189
0.3	0.04678
0.4	0.049133
0.5	0.000864
0.6	$2.56E-07$
0.7	$4.27E-13$
0.8	$1.64E-22$
0.9	$2.74E-40$

P	log(P(X))
0.1	−10.9348
0.2	−3.72366
0.3	−1.32994
0.4	−1.30863
0.5	−3.06356
0.6	−6.59137
0.7	−12.3692
0.8	−21.7855
0.9	−39.5621

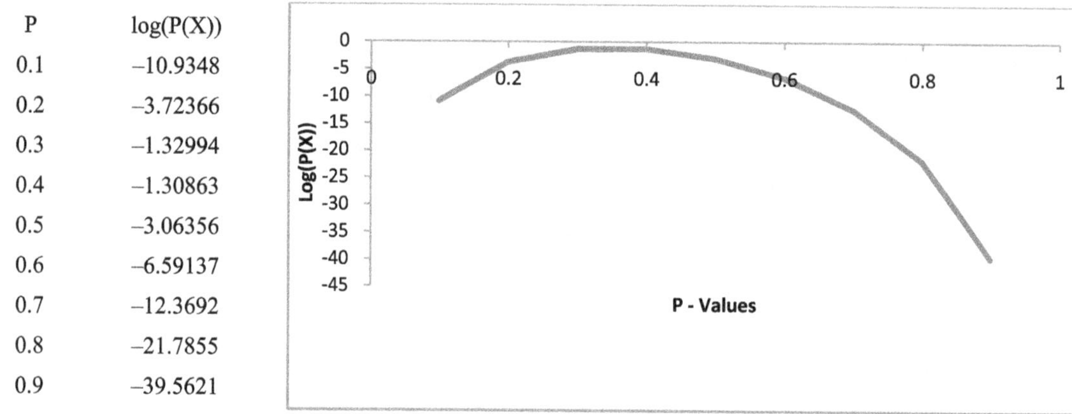

The maximum of the likelihood function occurs at the same value of P as the maximum of the likelihood function. In this example the plot of likelihood function against P and Log likelihood function against P the maximum value occurs when the value of P is 0.35.

The log likelihood is most useful function. The estimator of P defined by the value where (log) likelihood function takes its maximum is known as the maximum likelihood estimator of P. This function gives information about the precision of the estimator.

Cox-Regression

The Cox model, a regression method for survival data, provides an estimate of the hazard ratio and its confidence interval. The hazard ratio is an estimate of the ratio of the hazard rate in the treated versus the control group.

Cox regression (or proportional hazards regression) is method for investigating the effect of several variables upon the time when a specified event happens. The event or outcome can be considered as death, that is known as Cox regression for survival analysis. This Cox – regression model is used to verify risk scores developed from survival data, which allow for censoring.

A Cox model is a well-recognized statistical technique for exploring the relationship between the survival of a patient and several explanatory variables. The Cox Proportional – hazard model is essentially a regression model commonly used by statistician in medical research and it provides an estimate of the treatment effect on survival after adjustment for other explanatory variables. It also helps the investigator to estimate the hazard (or risk) of death, or other event of interest, for individuals, given their prognostic variables.

The Cox proportional-hazards model (Cox, 1972) is essentially a regression model commonly used statistical tools in medical research for verifying the association between the survival time of patients and one or more predictor variables.

Interpreting a Cox model involves examining the coefficients for each explanatory variable. A positive regression coefficient for an explanatory variable means that the hazard for patient having a high positive value on that particular variable is high. Conversely, a negative regression coefficient implies a better prognosis for patients with higher values of that variable.

Cox's method does not assume any particular distribution for the survival times, but it rather assumes that the effects of the different variables on survival are constant over time and are additive in a particular scale.

Since we are focusing mainly on relative hazard approach, in place of OR then the hazard function h(t) can be written as $h(t/X=x) = h(t/X = 0)e^{cx} = h_0(t)\ e^{cx}$ or it can be written as $\log(h(t)/X=x) = \log(h_0(t) + cx$, the function $h_0(t)$ is a base line hazard function when $X = 0$. The Coefficient c is taken as relative hazard due to increase in the level of variables X. If $c > 0$, e^c measures the increase value of hazard at all times t.

The Cox-Proportional hazards model produces a mathematical equation for the log hazard ratio as $h(t/X=x) = h(t/X = 0)e^{cx} = h_0(t)\ e^{c1x1\ +c2x2+........+ckxk,}$ after taking log both side then, we get

$$\log(h(t)/X=x) = \log(h_0(t) + c_1x_1 + c_2x_2 + c_3x_3 +--------------+c_kx_k$$

The first term depends only on time and the second one depends on X. We are only interested on the second term. If we estimate the only second term, a very important hypothesis has to be verified, that is called proportional hazards hypothesis. It means that the hazard ratio between two different observations does not depend on time. Using this we explain the effect of confounding, interactive, order and unordered categorical variables which are explained.

In case of Cox-Regression model, we are hiding the term intercept which will anchor down or reduce to estimate of risk.

When we go clinical investigation, there we find many situations, where several known quantities (or can be called as covariates), potentially they will affect prognosis of patient.

Example: Suppose two groups of patients are compared, those with and without a specific genotype. If one of the groups contains older subjects or individuals, any difference in survival may be attributable to genotype or age or indeed both. Hence when we are investigating survival in relation to any one factor, it is often desirable to adjust for the impact of others.

Cox proportional hazards model and hazard ratio.

The Cox model, a regression method for survival data, provides an estimate of the hazard ratio and its confidence interval. The hazard ratio is an estimate of the ratio of the hazard rate in the treated versus the control group.

Example: The data given in the table is about death of patients with an equal interval of time as shown in the table. Compute the hazard h(t), Hazard Rate (HR) and Ln(HR)

t	EVENTS(Death)	At Risk(Survivors)
0	0	10000
0.1	28	9972
0.2	58	9914
0.3	49	9865
0.4	64	9801
0.5	67	9734
0.6	91	9643
0.7	71	9572
0.8	115	9457

0.9	90	9367
1	113	9254
1.1	108	9146
1.2	89	9057
1.3	85	8972
1.4	122	8850
1.5	120	8730
1.6	116	8614
1.7	120	8494
1.8	138	8356
1.9	119	8237
2	134	8103

Solution:

t	EVENTS (Death)=d_i	At Risk(Survivors)=n_i	Hazard Estimate (h(t))= $e_i/n_i \times t_i$ or $h(t) = d_i/(n_i - 0.5e_i) \times u_i$	HR=$h(t_i)/(h(0))$	ln(HR)
0	0	10000	0	0	0
0.1	28	9972	0.028	2.08	0.73
0.2	58	9914	0.058	1.77	0.57
0.3	49	9865	0.050	2.32	0.84
0.4	64	9801	0.065	2.45	0.90
0.5	67	9734	0.069	3.35	1.21
0.6	91	9643	0.094	2.64	0.97
0.7	71	9572	0.074	4.32	1.46
0.8	115	9457	0.121	3.42	1.23
0.9	90	9367	0.096	4.33	1.47
1	113	9254	0.121	4.19	1.43
1.1	108	9146	0.117	3.49	1.25
1.2	89	9057	0.098	3.37	1.21
1.3	85	8972	0.094	4.89	1.59
1.4	122	8850	0.137	4.88	1.58
1.5	120	8730	0.137	4.78	1.56
1.6	116	8614	0.134	5.01	1.61
1.7	120	8494	0.140	5.85	1.77
1.8	138	8356	0.164	5.12	1.63
1.9	119	8237	0.143	5.86	1.77
2	134	8103	0.164		

$$h_0(t) = d_i/n_i \times t_i \ \ OR \ \ d_i/(n_i - 0.5e_i) \times u_i = 28/((10000 - 0.5 \times 28) \times 0.1) = 0.028$$

d_i = deaths , u_i = interval of time , n_i = Survivors

Similarly $h_1(t) = e_i/n_i \times t_i = 58/(9972 - 0.5 \times 58) \times 0.1 = 0.058$

$\qquad$ HR= $h_1(t)/h_0(t) = 0.058/0.028 = 2.07$

$\qquad$ HR = $e^b = 2.07$

$\qquad$ ln(HR) = $\ln(e^b) = b_1 = 0.73$

Similarly we can compute $b_2, b_3, \text{-------} b_i$

Basics of the Cox proportional hazards model

In case of this model, it is possible to evaluate simultaneously the effect of several factors on survival. In other way, we can say that, it allows us to examine how a particular factors which are going to influence the rate of a particular event happening (e.g getting a particular disease , death) at a particular point in time. This rate is commonly referred as the hazard rate. Predictor variables (or factors) are called as *covariates* in the survival-analysis.

The Cox model is written in the form of *hazard function* as by h(t). Briefly, the hazard function can be interpreted as the risk of dying at time t. The model expression can be written as $h(t) = h0(t) \times \exp(b_1x_1 + b_2x_2 + ... + b_nx_n)$

Where, t = the survival time, h(t) = the hazard function obtained using set of n covariates $(x_1, x_2, ..., x_n)$, the coefficients $(b_1, b_2, ..., b_n)$ measure the impact (i.e., the effect size) of covariates, the term h_0 is called the baseline hazard. It corresponds to the value of the hazard if all the xi are equal to zero (the quantity exp(0) equals 1). The 't' in h(t) reminds us that the hazard may vary over time.

The Cox model can be written as a multiple linear regression of the logarithm of the hazard on the variables xi, with the baseline hazard being an 'intercept' term that varies with time.

The quantities $\exp(b_i)$ are called hazard ratios (HR). A value of b_i greater than zero, or equivalently a hazard ratio greater than one, indicates that as the value of the ith covariate increases, the event hazard increases and thus the length of survival decreases. In another way, a hazard ratio above 1 indicates a covariate that is positively associated with the event probability, and thus negatively associated with the length of survival.

In summary,

$\qquad$ HR = 1: No effect

$\qquad$ HR < 1: Reduction in the hazard

$\qquad$ HR > 1: Increase in Hazard.

The estimated survival probability often called as the baseline survivor function, baseline values are {x} is evaluated at time t, where t is considered as time over a period of time. Time after 10 year may be considered time t for calculation of baseline survivor function. The base survival probability to the time t for the subjects who have mean values for all risk variable $x_1, x_2, x_3, \text{-----} x_n$ is written as $s(f, \bar{x})$

Use of the Cox Model in Trial of Disease duration

The hazard ratio derived from the Cox model does not translate directly into information about the duration of time until events. If the hazard ratio indicates a beneficial treatment effect, this implies that the time to the endpoint was reduced by treatment. However, as found in the clinical trial literature, the magnitude of the hazard ratio may be greater or less than the treatment benefit apparent from the median endpoint times. To compare these two statistics, the median endpoint time ratio can be calculated by dividing the control group median value by the treatment group median value. If there were a direct relationship between hazard ratio and median ratio, in a successful trial where the hazard ratio was 2, the median ratio would also be 2, indicating that the time to the endpoint in the treated group was half that of the control group.

Time at risk confound an exposure-disease relationship.

In the log rank test, stratification by time at risk can give explanation difference between the approaches of the Cox model and the logistic regression Model.

By applying proportional hazards model investigator can observe the controls for the effect of time at risk before going to measure the association between the risk factors and the outcome event, assuming that there will be no interaction between time at risk and the factors which are considered for the study.

In true sense the proportional hazards model that allows for the potential confounding effects of time at risk, but the logistic regression model does not explain the effect of time at risk.

In we are not considering such type of confounding, then both can be expected to yield similar results.

With the same procedure the investigator can anticipate different results when time at risk does confound an exposure of interest.

After analyzing the results of the data collected, both logistic regression and the Cox model provide differing fits, then the investigator can understand the effect of time at risk as a confounding variable.

In epidemiological study in order for confounding to occur, it is very much necessary to consider that.

1. time at risk be causally associated with outcome event
2. time at risk be associated with exposure.

In most of the epidemiological study the investigator expects the first of these conditions to hold.

But we cannot expect always that outcome event increases with time at risk.

Sometime this does hold good when time at risk is unrelated to the hazard (that is, the hazard function is constant).

When confounding by time at risk is considered, that hinges on the second condition, time at risk be associated with exposure.

Log-Rank test

The logrank test, or log-rank test, is a hypothesis test that will be used to compare the survival distributions of two samples. This test can be considered as a non-parametric test, which is more suitable to use when the data skewed right side more or skewed positively. It is one of the statistical method most widely used in clinical trials to establish the efficacy of a new treatment in comparison with a control treatment when the measurement is the time to event (The time from initial treatment to a heart attack or other events). The test is sometimes called the Mantel–Cox test, named after Nathan Mantel and David Cox. The log-rank test can also be called as a time-stratified Cochran–Mantel–Haenszel test.

The log-rank test statistic compares estimates of the hazard functions of the two groups at each observed event time. It is constructed by computing the observed and expected number of events in one of the groups at each observed event time and then adding these to obtain an overall summary across all-time points where there is an event.

Consider two groups with number of deaths and number of patients alive as listed in the 2×2 – contingency table

	Groups		
	Group 1	Group 2	Total
Number of deaths observed	a_i	b_i	$a_i + b_i$
Number of Patient alive	c_i	d_i	$C_i + d_i$
Total number of patients at risk	$a_i + c_i$	$b_i + d_i$	60

Methodology to calculate the Rank-test

1. Order the survival times until death for both groups combined, omitting censored times. Each time investigator will constitute a stratum for different time t_i

2. For each stratum obtain predicted frequency of the upper left-hand cell (For the variable a_i, corresponding predicted variable $e_i = ((a_i + b_i) \times (a_i + c_i))/ n_i$

3. v_i–variance for each is obtained using the equation $vi = (a_i + b_i)(c_i + d_i)(a_i + c_i)(b_i + d_i)/ n_i^2 \times (n_i - 1)$. Then the MH –test statistic λ_{MH}^2 is computed using the equation

$$\lambda_{MH}^2 = \frac{\left(\sum_{i=1}^{I} a_i - \sum_{i=1}^{I} e_i \right)^2}{\sum_{i=1}^{I} v_i}$$

4. The null hypothesis is rejected, and alternative hypothesis is accepted, when there is an association between disease and risk factor. This can be verified when the computed value of test statistics is greater than the tabulated value of Chi-square for the degree of freedom 1for the 5% or 1% level of significance.

Example:

	Groups		
	Group 1	Group 2	Total
Number of deaths observed	0	1	1
Number of Patient alive	25	13	38
Total number of patients at risk	25	14	39

Time	a_i	c_i	a_i+c_i	b_i	d_i	b_i+d_i	n_i	e_i	v_i
0	0	25	25	1	13	14	39	0.641	0.230
2	1	25	26	1	12	13	39	1.333	0.433
4	2	25	27	1	11	12	39	2.077	0.605
6	0	24	24	3	8	11	35	2.057	0.608
8	2	23	25	6	2	8	33	6.061	1.148
10	3	20	23	0	2	2	25	2.760	0.202
12	1	20	21	1	1	2	23	1.826	0.152
	9							16.755	3.379

$$\lambda^2_{MH} = \frac{\left(\sum_{i=1}^{I} a_i - \sum_{i=1}^{I} e_i\right)^2}{\sum_{i=1}^{I} v_i}$$

$$\lambda^2_{MH} = \frac{(9-16.755)^2}{3.379} = 17.80$$

Example: The data given below about the CHD event (outcome event) and body weight(Independent variable) of different category gives the detail about case group (no of subjects who got Disease) and the control group (number of subjects who did not get the disease). Compute Intercept and slopes for different category of body weight for the corresponding case and control group and fit the logistic regression model.

		CHD Event		
		Case - Disease (D)	Control -NO Disease	Total
	<=140	30 a_1	550 b_1	580
Body Weight (lb)	x_1=140-150	35 a_2	500 b_2	535
	x_2=150-160	60 a_3	600 b_3	660
	x_3=160-170	70 a_4	510 b_4	580
	x_4 =>170	90 a_5	750 b_5	840
	Total	285	2910	3195

	Equation to Compute probability value of an event	Probability	Equation to obtain Intercept and Slopes	Incept and Slopes
	$\ln((a_1/c_1)/(b_1/c_1))$	$-2.91 = P_0$	$a = P_0$	-2.91
Computation of	$\ln((a_2/c_2)/(b_2/c_2))$	$-2.66 = P_1$	$b_1 = P_1 - P_0$	0.25
Intercept and	$\ln((a_3/c_3)/(b_3/c_3))$	$-2.30 = P_2$	$b_2 = P_2 - P_0$	0.61
Slopes	$\ln((a_4/c_4)/(b_4/c_4))$	$-1.99 = P_3$	$b_3 = P_3 - P_0$	0.92
	$\ln((a_5/c_5)/(b_5/c_5))$	$-2.12 = P_4$	$b_4 = P_4 - P_0$	0.79

The logistic regression model is $\text{Log}(Px/1 - Px) = a + b_1x_1 + b_2x_2 + b_3x_3 + b_4x_4$

$$= -2.91 + 0.25 \times x_1 + 0.61 \times x_2 + 0.92 \times x_3 + 0.79 \times x_4$$

Example: In a sample of 600 subjects chosen from a population are, the subjects are stratified into different subgroups on the basis of different factor like age, smoking habit, consumption of alcohol and outcome event (Coronary heart disease). The data is as listed in the below.

Risk Factor (Smoking)	CHD(Yes)	CHD (No) Control	Total
AGE<50			
Exposure	35	45	80
Non Exposure	10	30	40
Total	45	75	120

Risk Factor (Smoking)	CHD(Yes)	CHD (No) Control	Total
AGE -50 -60			
Exposure	50	70	120
Non Exposure	20	50	70
	70	120	190

Risk Factors (Interaction of Smoking and Consumption of Alcohol)	CHD(Yes) (Case)	CHD (No) (Control)	Total
AGE ≥ 60 Exposure-both	70	120	190
Non Exposure-both	30	60	90
	100	180	280

Third strata is due to interaction effect of smoking and consumption of alcohol. Obtain multiple logistic regression model.

Solution:

Risk Factor (Smoking)	CHD(Yes)	CHD (No) Control	Total
AGE<50			
Exposure	35-a$_1$	45-b$_1$	80
Non Exposure	10-c$_1$	30-d$_1$	40
Total	45	75	120
Risk Factor (Smoking)	CHD(Yes) CHD(Yes)	CHD (No) CHD (No)	Total
	Case	Control	

AGE -50 -60

Exposure	50	70	120
Non Exposure	20	50	70
	70	120	190

Risk Factors (Interaction of Smoking and Consumption of Alcohol)	CHD(Yes) (Case)	CHD (No) (Control)	Total
AGE $\geq$ 60 Exposure-both	70	120	190
Non Exposure-both	30	60	90
	100	180	280

$P_0 = a_1/80 = 35/80 = 0.4375$

Age <50 is confounder and Smoking is risk Factor $= x0$

$a_0 = \ln(P_0/(1 - P_0)) = \ln(0.4375/(1 - 0.4375)) = -0.2513$

$P_1 = a_2/120 = 50/120 = 0.4167$

$\ln(P_1/(1 - P_1)) = \ln(0.4167/(1 - 0.4167)) = -0.3365$

$b_1 = \ln(P_1/(1 - P_1)) - \ln(P_0/(1 - P_0)) = -0.3365 - (-0.2513) = -0.0852$

Age 50-60 is confounder and Smoking is risk Factor $= x_1$

$P_2 = a_3/120 = 70/190 = 0.3684$

$\ln(P_2/(1 - P_2)) = \ln(0.3684/(1 - 0.3684)) = -0.5389$

$b_2 = \ln(P_2/(1 - P_2)) - \ln(P_0/(1 - P_0)) = -0.5389 - (-0.2513) = -0.2877$

Age> 60 is confounder and Smoking & alcohol consumption (interaction Factors) are risk Factor $= x_2 \times z$

$x_2 =$ Smoking and $z =$ alcohol ($x_2 Z$- Interaction)

Then the logistic regression equation is $y = a_0 + b_1 x_1 + b_2 x_2 z$

$y = -0.2513 - 0.2877 x_1 - 0.2877 x_2 z$

What is matching in epidemiology?

We have learned how to adjust the confounding variables during the analysis in the epidemiological investigation. The type of adjustment to be made at the designing stage by the process of matching is the most common. Matching is one in each case is matched with a single control. Matching is not uncommon in epidemiological studies and refers to the selection of unexposed subjects of controls with certain important characteristics which are very much identical to cases. This could be done by matching controls with case.

For example, we might match the sex of the control to the sex of the case. The idea in matching is to match upon a potential confounding variable in order to remove the confounding effect.

Matching

The most common matching type is one in which each case is matched with a single control. (1: 1 matching or Pair matching), so that control can have identical (or at least very similar) values of confounding variable. In this type of design, both case-control are balance identically, so that any difference between them cannot be due to confounder.

In general, common matching variables, the investigator would like to choose are age and sex. In particular circumstances race, marital status, hospital, time of admission to the hospital, blood group and social class are some matching criteria. Generally, the continuous variable, such as age, are matched within a predetermined range. Sometimes this is done by grouping the variables, such that the age can be categorized into 5-years age groups and control must be within the same 5-years age group as the case. The finer the grouping are, the more effective the matching.

There are two common misconceptions about case-control studies, that matching in itself eliminates (controls) confounding by the matching factors, and that if matching has been performed, then a "matched analysis" is required. However, matching in a case-control study does not control for confounding by the matching factors; in fact, it can introduce confounding by the matching factors even when it does not exist in the source population. Thus, a matched design may require controlling for the matching factors in the analysis. However, it is not the case that a matched design requires a matched analysis. Provided that there are no problems of sparse data, control for the matching factors can be obtained, with no loss of validity and a possible increase in precision, using a "standard" (unconditional) analysis, and a "matched" (conditional) analysis may not be required or appropriate.

Principles of Matching

Confounder implies that the confounding factor (one of the exposures) is not evenly distributed between cases and controls. Therefore in order to overcome the problem of confounding the simplest method is to design a study in which cases and controls (or exposed and unexposed) would have an equal distribution of the confounding factor. This process is called matching.

Matching is most often applied into case controls studies, however matching may be performed also in cohort studies.

We usually identify two types of matching process, Individual matching and frequency matching have the same consequence, and the matching will be taken into account during the analysis.

Frequency Matching

In the process of matching, matching not done individually but it is done for groups of subjects. In such case investigator selects a group subjects of controls which is matched to a group of cases with respect to a particular characteristic (that may be a confounding factor).

For example, when we select a case-control study with 40 cases where are 15 men and 25 women, in the same we would select control group having the same gender distribution. We would first select 15 men from the male study population and then 25 women from the female study population to match the frequency. It is more important to balance the sample size to achieve our objective of frequency matching.

The impact of frequency matching very instantaneous for the data chosen for analysis. In Case-Control study it is not possible to compute the conditional probabilities, $P(D/E)$ or $P(E/\overline{D})$ due to the manipulation of sample sizes against the matching factor C and it modifies the observed frequency of exposure in cases and controls.   But it is possible to calculate the, $P(D/E, C = c_i)$ or $P(E/D, C=c_i)$, where c_i denotes the particular level of the matching variable C. With this process it is possible to estimate the Odd Ratio associating E and D after making the stratification of C.

This frequency matching uses only a few distinct levels of the matching factors, so that this stratification can be used to examine the relationship between E and D.

Why Matching

Matching controls to cases is nothing but stratifying in advance of analysis or strata is done before the study has to be done during the selection of controls. When we select one control per case, each stratum will include one case and one control. Then it is possible to have as many strata as pairs in the study. The main focus of matching is to prepare the analysis. Matching optimizes the number of cases and controls per stratum. It also can help us to avoid for having no case or no control in a stratum, as could happen when doing a stratified analysis afterwards (The biggest inefficiency in a stratified analysis done afterward would occur when in a stratum there is either no case or no control). This helps us to improve the efficiency of an analysis by distributing cases and controls between strata in a better way.

Concordant and discordant pairs

Use of concordant and discordant pairs to describe the relationship between pairs of observations. To calculate the concordant and discordant pairs, the data are treated as ordinal, so ordinal data should be appropriate for our application. The number of concordant and discordant pairs are used in calculations for Kendall's tau, which measures the association between two ordinal variables.

The procedure for calculating concordant and discordant pairs compares the classifications for two variables (for example, X and Y) on the same two items. If the direction of classifications is the same, the pairs are concordant. For example, both X and Y rate item 1 higher than item 2. If the direction of the classification is not the same, the pair is discordant. For example, X rates item 1 higher than item 2 but Y rates item 1 lower than item 2.

Specifically, there are a pair of observations $- (X_i, Y_i)$ and (X_j, Y_j):

The pair is concordant if $X_i > X_j$ and $Y_i > Y_j$ or $X_i < X_j$ and $Y_i < Y_j$

The pair is discordant if $X_i > X_j$ and $Y_i < Y_j$ or $X_i < X_j$ and $Y_i > Y_j$

For example, suppose a group of friends are playing darts. They identify their skill level as beginner, intermediate, or expert, and collect data on their accuracy - low, medium, and high.

Skill	Low	Med	High
Beginner	10	2	1
Intermediate	3	5	5
Expert	3	7	3

A pair of observations is concordant if the subject who is higher on one variable is also higher on the other variable. A pair of observations is discordant if the subject who is higher on one variable is lower on the other variable.

Number of concordant pairs:

- Beginner, Low * Intermediate, Med = 50
- Beginner, Low * Expert, Med = 70
- Beginner, Low * Intermediate, High = 50
- Beginner, Low * Expert, High= 30
- Beginner, Med * Intermediate, High = 10
- Beginner, Med * Expert, High = 6
- Intermediate, Low * Expert, Med = 21
- Intermediate, Low * Expert, High = 9
- Intermediate, Med * Expert, High = 15

Number of discordant pairs:

Intermediate, Low * Beginner, Med = 6

Intermediate, Low * Beginner, High = 3

Expert, Low * Intermediate, Med = 15

Expert, Low * Intermediate, High = 15

Expert, Low * Beginner, Med = 6

Expert, Low * Beginner, High = 3

Expert, Med * Beginner, High = 7

Expert, Med * Intermediate, High = 35

Intermediate, Med * Beginner, High = 5

Concordance. The amount of similarity in phenotype between a set of individuals. May be used to refer to the presence of the same trait in both members of a pair of twins.

"Concordance is a new approach to the prescribing and taking of medicines. It is an agreement reached after negotiation between a patient and a healthcare professional that respects the beliefs and wishes of the patient in determining whether, when, and how medicines are to be taken."

Pairs with the same exposure status for both case and control are called as concordant pairs, the total number of concordant pairs is $c_1 + c_2 = c$. The pairs with different exposures are called as discordant, then there will be $d_1 + d_2 = d$ discordant pairs.

Analysis of Matched Studies

When a case-control is matched, the analysis must take account of matching, instead of unmatched analysis, where the odd ratio (OR) will tend to be very close to unity, hence we may find some mistakes in finding the effect of risk factor. This method will reduce, because both cases and controls will be more are similar to each other, than they would have been, when independent sampling is adopted. This technique is restricted to 2×2 table or combination of such tables.

Results of paired Case-Control study can be written as

	Control Exposed to Risk factor	
Case exposed to Risk Factor	**Yes**	**No**
Yes	A	B
No	C	D

Here A and D are considered as concordant and C and B are considered as discordant group.

1:1 Matching

In this case the subjects will be classified into exposure / not exposure to the risk factor of interest, that data should be presented in the form of the study pairs. Each subjects of the pair is either exposed or not exposed to the risk factor and either a case pair or control, will give, four possible outcomes like A, D and B , C as shown in the table. Pairs with the same exposure status for both case and control are called as concordant pairs, the total number of concordant pairs is A + D.

Pairs with different exposures are called as discordant, there are B + C discordant pairs.

Let P be the be the probability of discordant pair, which has an exposed case, then $\hat{P} = \dfrac{B}{B+C}$.

When the Null Hypothesis is considered, that indicates there will be no association between the risk factor and event of disease. Each discordant pair is just as likely to have the case exposed as to have control exposed.

Then the null hypothesis can be written as H0: $\hat{P} = \frac{1}{2}$

This is one of the test for the value of proportion. Then we can use the equation $\dfrac{P - P_0}{\sqrt{P_0(1-P_0)}}$

Substituting the value in the equation we get, $\dfrac{\dfrac{B}{B+C} - \dfrac{1}{2}}{\sqrt{1/2\left(1-\dfrac{1}{2}\right)/(B+C)}}$

After simplifying and Squaring we get $\dfrac{(B+C)^2}{(B+C)}$

Then we compare to the Chi-square value for DOF 1 using continuity corrected Chi-Square statistics

$$\frac{\left(2d_1 - d\right)^2}{d} \qquad\qquad .....(9.3)$$

$$d1 = B, \; d = B + C$$

This is based on McNamara's test, the test for no association in a paired study Proportions.

To obtain OR we use $\;\; OR = \dfrac{\hat{P}}{1 - \hat{P}}$

By applying the equation 1 and 2 we get $OR = \dfrac{B}{C}$ because $B + C \approx C$

In case of Paired Case-Control studies, $B + C$ will be small, and it is required to use exact limits for OR. They are written (OR_L, OR_U).

$$OR_L = \frac{B}{(C+1)FL} \;\; \text{ and } \;\; OR_U = \frac{(B+1)Fu}{C}$$

Fl and Fu are the upper $2\dfrac{1}{2}$ point of F on $(2(C + 1), 2B)$ and $(2(B + 1), 2C)$ DOF 1 respectively.

Mantel-Haenszel Techniques Applied to Pair-Matched

The matched paired data for case-control can be written in four possible ways as

Both Case-Control are exposed for the risk factor

		CONTROL		
		Exposed (E)	Not Exposed ($\bar{E}$)	Total
Case	Exposed	X		
	Not Exposed ($\overline{E}$)			
	Total			

In this study Case exposed and Control is not exposed for the risk factor

		CONTROL		
		Exposed (E)	**Not Exposed ($\bar{E}$)**	**Total**
Case	Exposed		X	
	Not Exposed ($\bar{E}$)			
	Total			

In this study Case is not exposed and Control is exposed for the risk factor

		CONTROL		
Case		**Exposed (E)**	**Not Exposed ($\overline{E}$)**	**Total**
	Exposed(E)			
	Not Exposed ($\overline{E}$)	X		
	Total			

In this study both Case and Control are not exposed for the risk factor

		CONTROL		
Case		**Exposed (E)**	**Not Exposed ($\overline{E}$)**	**Total**
	Exposed(E)			
	Not Exposed ($\overline{E}$)		X	
	Total			

1:1 Matching

If the matching pair is 1:1, the exposure patterns in the four types of matched pairs can be written as

1.

		CONTROL		
Case		**Exposed (E)**	**Not Exposed ($\overline{E}$)**	**Total**
	Exposed	1	1	2
	Not Exposed ($\overline{E}$)	0	0	0
	Total	1	1	2

2.

		CONTROL		Total
Case		**Exposed (E)**	**Not Exposed ($\overline{E}$)**	
	Exposed	1	0	1
	Not Exposed ($\overline{E}$)	0	1	1
	Total	1	1	2

3.

		CONTROL		Total
Case		**Exposed (E)**	**Not Exposed ($\overline{E}$)**	
	Exposed	0	1	1
	Not Exposed ($\overline{E}$)	1	0	1
	Total	1	1	2

4.

		CONTROL		Total
Case		**Exposed (E)**	**Not Exposed ($\overline{E}$)**	
	Exposed	0	0	0
	Not Exposed ($\overline{E}$)	1	1	2
	Total	1	1	2

By applying the respective equation $E(a_i)$ and V_i have to be obtained. The mathematical equation used to compute predicted or expected values is $E(a_i) = A_{ii} = (a_i + b_i)(a_i + c_i) / n_i$ and the equation used to compute variance $V_i = ((a_i + b_i)(c_i + d_i)(a_i + c_i)(b_i + d_i) / n_i^2(n_i - 1)$

Then $\qquad A_1 = (1+1)(1+0)/2 = 2 \times \dfrac{1}{2} = 1$

$$A_2 = (1+0)(1+0)/2 = \dfrac{1}{2}$$

$$A_3 = (0+1)(0+1)/2 = \dfrac{1}{2}$$

$$A_4 = (0+0)(1+1)/2 = 0$$

Then $\qquad V_1 = ((1+1)(0+0)(1+0)(1+0)) / 2^2(2-1) = 0$

$$V_2 = ((1+0)(0+1)(1+0)(0+1)) / 2^2(2-1) = \dfrac{1}{4}$$

Similarly, $\qquad V_3 = \dfrac{1}{4}$ and $V_4 = 0$

By applying Cochran-Mantel-Haenszel test statistic and Mantel-Haenszel odds ratio, the values can be written in a table as shown below.

Pair Types	Name	a_i	A_i	V_i	a_id_i/n_i	b_ic_i/n_i
1	A	1	1	0	0	0
2	B	1	$\dfrac{1}{2}$	1/4	1/2	0
3	C	0	$\dfrac{1}{2}$	1/4	0	½
4	D	0	0	0	0	0

$\Sigma a_i = A + B$, because $A = 1$ $B = 1$

$\Sigma A_i = A + B/2 + C/2 + 0 = A + ((B+C)/2)$

$\Sigma V_i = 0 + B/4 + C/4 + 0 = (B+C)/4$

$\Sigma \dfrac{a_id_i}{n_i} = 0 + B/2 + 0 + 0 = B/2$

$\Sigma \dfrac{b_ic_i}{n_i} = 0 + 0 + C/2 + 0 = C/2$

According to Cochran-Mantel-Haenszel Test we get $\lambda^2_{CMH} = \dfrac{\left(\Sigma a_i - \Sigma A_i\right)^2}{V_i}$

$$= \dfrac{\left[(A+B) - A + \dfrac{B+C}{2}\right]^2}{\dfrac{B+C}{4}}$$

$$= \dfrac{(B-C)^2}{B+C}$$

For unmatched data, there will be bias in small sample for the computation of Odds Ratio, and it is obtained by the equation $\hat{OR}_{SS} = \dfrac{B}{C+1}$

1:2 matching

In this situation the control will be to 2 (C = 2) all strata's are of same size 3 (1 case and 2 control) in each group. In this case 2(C + 1) = 6 and different 2×2 table can be constructed

Woolf's Method for Adjusted Odds Ratio

1. No exposure

	CONTROL		
Case	**Exposed (E)**	**Not Exposed** $(\overline{E})$	Total
Exposed(E)	0	0	0
Not Exposed ($\overline{E}$)	1	2	3
Total	1	2	3

2. One exposure

	CONTROL		
Case	**Exposed (E)**	**Not Exposed** $(\overline{E})$	**Total**
Exposed(E)	1	0	1
Not Exposed ($\overline{E}$)	0	2	2
Total	1	2	3

	CONTROL		**Total**
Case	**Exposed (E)**	**Not Exposed** $(\overline{E})$	
Exposed(E)	0	1	1
Not Exposed ($\overline{E}$)	1	1	2
Total	1	2	3

3. Two exposures

		CONTROL		Total
		Exposed (E)	**Not Exposed ($\overline{E}$)**	
Case	Exposed(E)	1	1	2
	Not Exposed ($\overline{E}$)	0	1	1
	Total	1	2	3

		CONTROL		Total
		Disease (D)	**No Disease ($\overline{D}$)**	
Case	Exposed(E)	0	2	2
	Not Exposed ($\overline{E}$)	1	0	1
	Total	1	2	3

4.

		CONTROL		Total
		Exposed (E)	**Not Exposed ($\overline{E}$)**	
Case	Exposed(E)	1	2	3
	Not Exposed ($\overline{E}$)	0	0	0
	Total	1	2	3

The matched process helps us to control for variables that may confound our results. If we match out cases and controls on a separate variable, then we can see if there is a difference based just on the exposure. There we can have 4 potential outcomes when we can make the pairs of cases and controls. They can be classified as

1. Case exposed – Control exposed (EE)
2. Case exposed – Control Not exposed (EN)
3. Case Not exposed – Control exposed (NE)
4. Case not exposed – Control not exposed (NN)

By applying the respective equation $E(a_i)$ and V_i have to be obtained. The mathematical equation used to compute predicted or expected values is $E(a_i) = A_{ii} = (a_i + b_i)(a_i + c_i) / n_i$ and the equation used to compute variance $V_i = ((a_i + b_i)(c_i + d_i)(a_i + c_i)(b_i + d_i) / n_i^2(n_i - 1)$

Then $\quad A_1 = (0 + 1)(0 + 0)/3 = 1 \times \dfrac{0}{3} = 0$

$A_2 = (1 + 0)(1 + 0)/3 = \dfrac{1}{2}$

$A_3 = (1 + 0)(1 + 1)/3 = \dfrac{2}{3}$

$A_4 = (1 + 0)(1 + 2)/3 = 1$

Then
$$V_1 = ((0 + 1)(0 + 2)(0 + 0)(0 + 3))/3^2 (3 - 1) = 0$$

$$V_2 = ((1 + 0)(0 + 2)(1 + 0)(0 + 2))/3^2 (3 - 1) = \frac{2}{9}$$

Similarly
$$V_3 = \frac{2}{9} \text{ and } V_4 = 0$$

By applying Cochran-Mantel-Haenszel test statistic and Mantel-Haenszel odds ratio, the values can be written in a table as shown below.

Pair Types	Name	a_i	A_i	V_i	$a_i d_i / n_i$	$b_i c_i / n_i$
1	A	0	0	0	0	0
2	B	1	$\frac{1}{3}$	2/9	2/3	0
3	C	1	2/3	2/9	1/3	0
4	D	1	0	0	0	0

$\Sigma a_i = B + C + D$, because $B = 1$ $C = 1$, $D = 1$

$\Sigma A_i = B/3 + 2C/3 = ((B + 2C)/3)$

$\Sigma V_i = 0 + 2B/9 + 2C/9 + 0 = (2B + 2C)/9 = (B + C)2/9$

$$\Sigma \frac{a_i d_i}{n_i} i = 0 + 2B/3 + C/3 + 0 = (2B + C)/3$$

$$\Sigma \frac{b_i c_i}{n_i} i = 0 + 0 + 0 + 0 = 0$$

According to Cochran-Mantel-Haenszel Test we get $\lambda^2_{CMH} = \dfrac{\left(\Sigma a_i - \Sigma A_i\right)^2}{V_i}$

Again the data can be separated into Discordant pairs and Concordant pairs

CONCORDANT PAIRS	Case exposed – Control exposed (EE) - a
	Case not exposed – Control not exposed (NN) - d
DISCORDANT PAIRS	Case exposed – Control Not exposed (EN) - b
	Case Not exposed – Control exposed (NE) - c

CASE-CONTROL PAIRS

		CONTROL	
		Exposed	**Not Exposed**
CASE	Exposed	a	b
	Unexposed	c	d

Computation of Odds ratio is based on discordant pairs.

$$\text{Odds Ratio (Matched Pair)} = \frac{b}{c}$$

Example: Data listed in the table is about matched pair case-control study on spontaneous abortions and coronary heart disease between the married and unmarried women who are chosen from the study population.

		Control		
		≥1 SA	**No. SA**	
Case	≥ SA	12	18	30
	No SA	5	25	30
		17	43	60

Compute McNemar's test value and verify the level of association between Spontaneous abortion and CHD of the subjects chosen for study.

Solution:

The equation used for the computation of McNemar's test value is $\lambda^2_{CMH} = \dfrac{(B-C)^2}{B+C} = 4.83$

The standard value of Chi-square test value $= \lambda^2$ is equal to 3.84 for the degree of freedom 1. Calculated value is greater than standard value, hence there is strong evidence to say the effect of Spontaneous abortion and CHD between the married and un-married women.

Difference between Hazard Ratios and Risk Ratios (or Relative Risk)

Hazard ratio can be considered as risk ratio or relative risk at each moment of time, but technically they are not same. However HR helps us to understand what is happening to the population at that particular time, which is considered by an investigator.

Like Hazard ratio, risk ratio or relative risk does not give more stress for timings of the event, but it gives more preference for the occurrence of the event at the end of the study.

In general, hazard ratio takes account or considers not only of the total number of events, but also of the timing of each event.

CHAPTER 10

Graphs

The theoretical meaning of graph is the pictorial representation of data which has been collected and tabulated in table. Graphs are used to convey the general patterns in a set of observations at a single glance. The frequency distribution graphs are designed to reveal more effectively the characteristic features of a frequency data. Such types of graphs are more appealing to the eye and are more perceptible to the mind than the data which are written in table or convincing, appealing and easily understood method of presenting the statistical data is the use of graph. In general, graphs can help to clarify the public health problems. Graphs are helpful in finding patterns, trends, aberrations, similarities, and differences in data. They are useful for effectively describing and communicating health-related events according to person, place and time. The building blocks of graphs are numbers, ratios, proportions and rates.

A graph is an ideal way of presenting data to others. In epidemiology, presenter will have two scales or axes, one horizontal and one vertical, that intersect at a right angle. The horizontal axis is known as the x-axis and that will be used represent the of the independent (or x) variable, such as time or age group. The vertical axis is the y-axis will be used represent the dependent (or y) variable, which, in epidemiology investigator makes the frequency measure such as number of cases or rate of disease. Each axis should be labeled to show the both the names of the variables and the units in which the variables are measured on the both the axes also be mentioned on the line.

An alternative approach to this problem of incompatible scales is to use a **logarithmic transformation** for the y-axis, which is termed as a **"semi-log" graph**, this technique is useful for displaying a variable with a wide range of values. The x-axis uses the arithmetic-scale, but the y-axis is measured on a logarithmic scale in place of arithmetic scale. As a result, the distance from 1 to 10 on the y- axis is the same as the distance from 10 to 100 or 100 to 1,000.

A graph can be defined as a two dimensional drawing showing relationship between two sets of information or numbers using a line , curve, series of bars, other symbols in a simple and compact format.

Histogram, Bar diagram, Frequency Polygon, Frequency curve, Ogive, Semilog graph, Pie chart, g. Stem and leaf graph etc.

Histogram

It is one of the most popular and commonly used device for constructing graph of continuous frequency distribution. This is one of the useful presentation of a frequency table.

The frequency or proportion of observations in each class-interval is plotted as a rectangle. For the construction of Histogram, class-interval should be of equal width. Each class-interval drawn on X-axis and by a section (base of the rectangle) which is equal to the magnitude of the class-interval. On each class-interval (as base) series of rectangles are erected with corresponding frequency of each interval as height of rectangles. The series of adjacent rectangles (one for each class) so formed gives the histogram of the frequency distribution and its area represents the total frequency of the distribution as distributed throughout the different classes.

The choice of interval for histogram depends on the nature of data, the distribution of data and what purpose we are presenting the data in the form of graph.

The histogram is very commonly used graph in epidemiology to reflect the frequency of health-related outcomes or outcomes over time. This graph shows course of a disease outbreak is named as epidemic curve. The overall shape of the epidemic curve can reveal the extent to which the events and exposures are associated.

Example: The frequency distribution of heights of 30 patients in centimeter is as listed below. Construct histogram for the given data.

Height in cms Class – Interval		Number of Patients f
139	149	6
149	159	9
159	169	7
169	179	5
179	189	2
189	199	1
		30

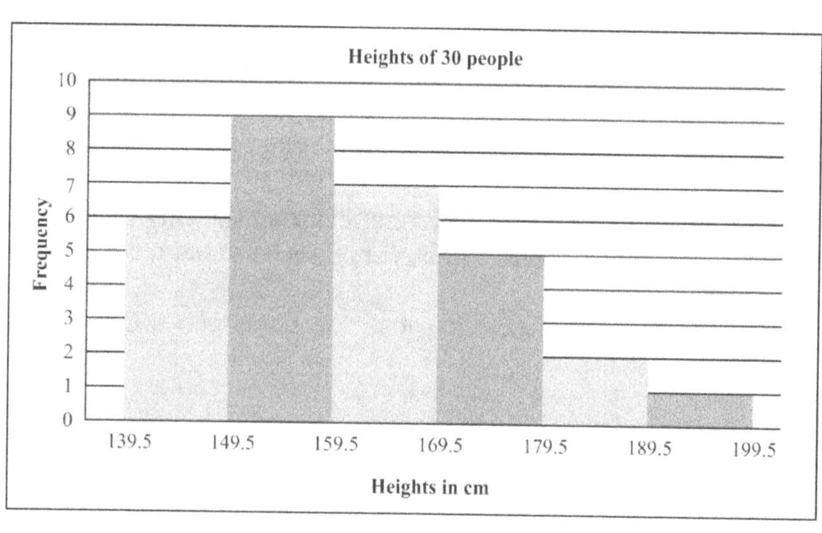

***Example*:** The frequency distribution of 500 patients. Construct histogram for the given data.

CLASS - INTERVAL	Frequency
−3.5 to −2.51	9
−2.5 to −1.51	32
−1.5 to −0.51	109
−0.5 to 0.49	180
0.5 to 1.49	132
1.5 to 2.49	34
2.5 to 3.49	4
	500

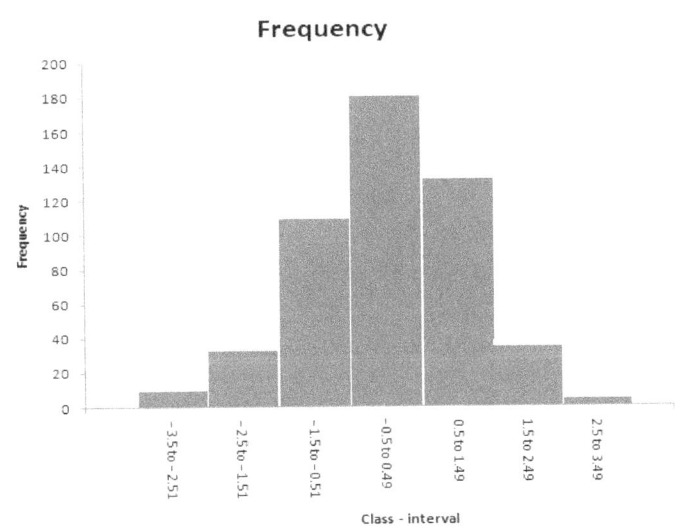

Pie Charts

Pie Charts are popular ways of presenting categorical data. The pie or circle represents 100% or all of the results. Here circle will be divided into different sections or segments, they are also called as sectors representing certain proportions or percentage of various component parts to the total. Such a sub-divided circle diagram is known as **Pie-chart.**

These charts are frequently used in epidemiology study to present the **Proportional mortality** ratio and death-to case ratio effectively in appropriate circumstances.

The proportional mortality ratio is the number of deaths from a specific cause in a specific time per 100 deaths from all causes during the same period.

The death to case ratio is the number of deaths attributed to a particular disease during a specified time period divided by the number of new cases of that disease identified during the same period.

***Example* 1:** Data given below is about the Absolute and relative frequencies of acne scar in 18-year-old adolescents (n = 2.414). Construct Pie chart for this data.

Prevalence	Absolute frequency (n)	Relative frequencies
NO	1855	76.84
YES	559	23.16
Total	2414	100

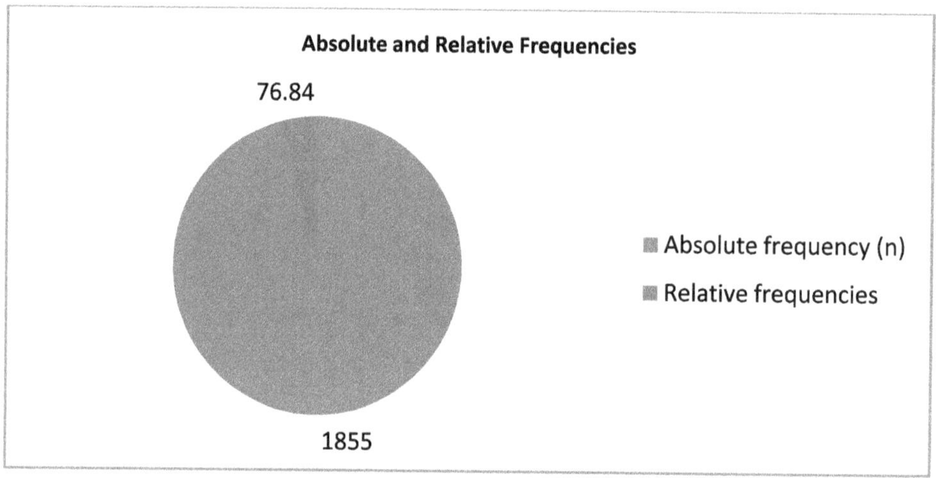

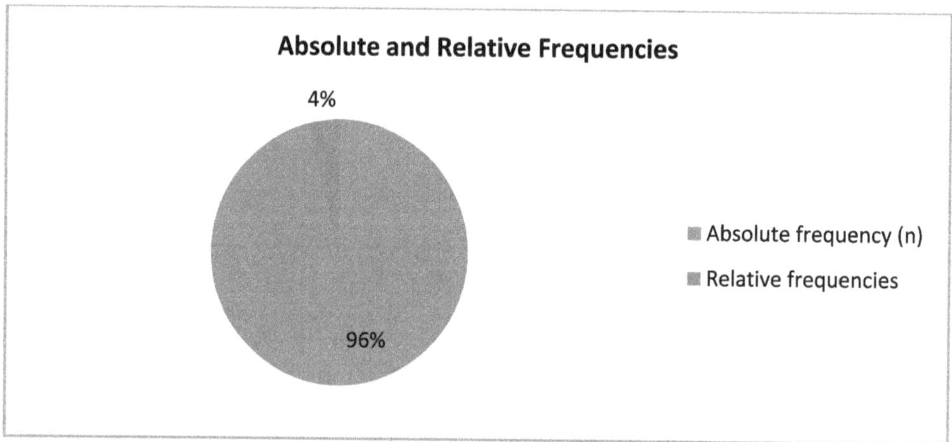

***Example* 2:** Data collected by an investigator about the number patients in all states of south india who are affected by HIV in a particular year is as listed below. Construct the Pie-Chart for the given data.

State	Number of HIV Patients	Percent
Karnataka	3600	14.0625
Kerala	5000	19.53125
Andhra Pradesh	7000	27.34375
Tamil Nadu	6000	23.4375
Telengaana	4000	15.625

Solution:

State	Number of HIV Patients	Percent
Karnataka	3600	14.0625
Kerala	5000	19.53125
Andhra Pradesh	7000	27.34375
Tamil Nadu	6000	23.4375
Telengana	4000	15.625
	25600	

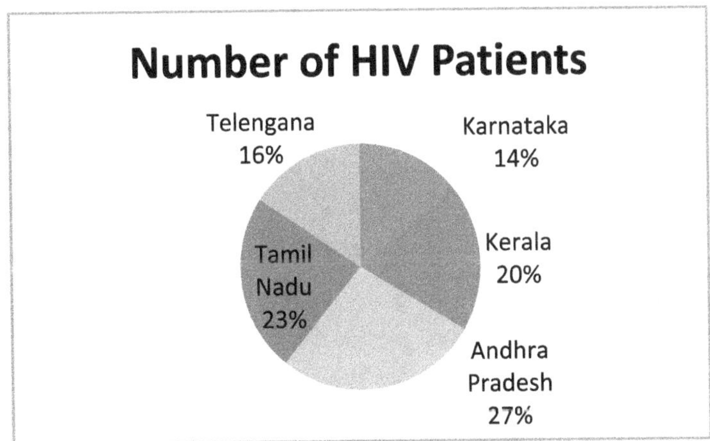

Bar Chart

Bar diagram is one of the simplest bar chart is used to display the data from a one-variable table where each value or category of the variable is represented by a bar. Hence this graph is most satisfactory for categorical data or series. The length of the bar is proportional to the number of persons or events in that category. Variables shown in bar charts are either discrete and non-continuous (e.g., race; sex) or are treated as though they were discrete and non-continuous (e.g., age groups rather than age intervals on the axis). Bars can be presented either horizontally or vertically. The length or height of each bar is proportional to the frequency of the event in that category. For this reason, a scale break should not be used with a bar chart since this could lead to misinterpretation in comparing the magnitude of different categories. A vertical bar chart differs from a histogram. In this method each bars are separated, but in case of histogram bars are joined.

This distinction follows from the type of variable used on the x-axis. A histogram is used to show the frequency distribution of a continuous variable such as age or serum cholesterol or dates of onset during an epidemic.

Example: The data given in the table is about the distribution SBP of male and female patients along with multiple risk factors like cardiovascular disease and diabetes etc. Construct Bar graph for the given data.

SBP	Number Male Patients	Number of Female Patients
<110	20	15
110-119	50	26
120-129	111	80
130-139	90	75
140-149	60	50
150-159	45	40
160-169	30	25
170-179	20	15
≥180	10	5

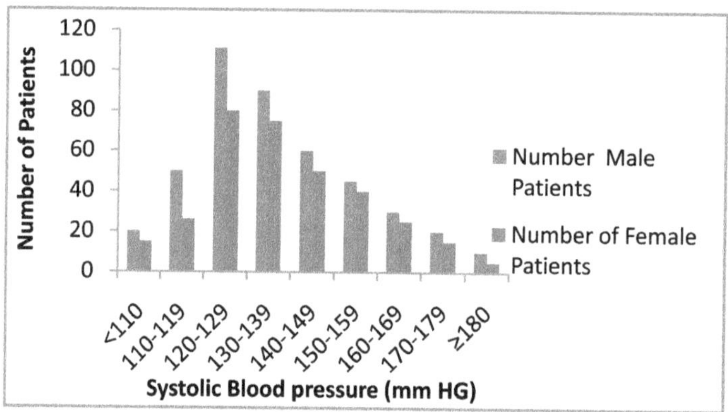

Example: The following data shows the number of deaths due to different diseases in a particular year. Construct simple Bar – chart or Diagram

Disease	Number of deaths
Cancer	100
Ulcer	200
CHD	250
ASTHAM	300
Juandice	150

Construct Bar – Chart or Diagram.

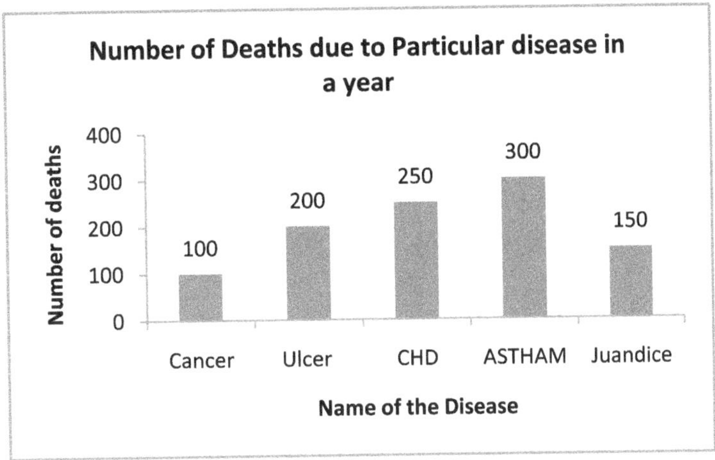

Example: In a group of 54 patients, who were suffering from knee pain due to Osteoarthritis problem and these 54 patients or subjects were divided into three groups consisting of 18 patients to each group and they were treated with Ozone , PRA and 25% dextrose . Construct bar chart for the data given below.

Age	OZONE	PRA	25% DEXTROSE	Total
40-50	5	10	4	19
50-60	3	5	8	16
60-70	10	3	6	19
Total	18	18	18	54

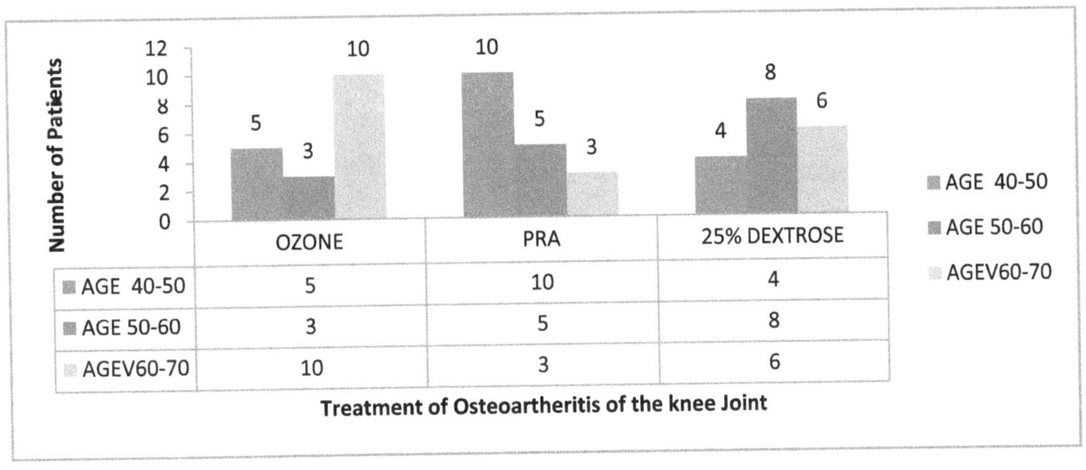

	OZONE	PRA	25% DEXTROSE
AGE 40-50	5	10	4
AGE 50-60	3	5	8
AGEV60-70	10	3	6

Line Graph

A line graph is a graphical representation of data that changes continuously over period of time. A line graph may also be referred to as a line chart. Within a line graph, there are points connecting the data to show a continuous change. The lines in a line graph can descend and ascend based on the data.

Each variable is plotted along an axis. They are good at showing specific values of data, meaning that gives that one variable determined by other variable easily. They show trends in data clearly, meaning that their visibly show how one variable is affected by the other as it increases or decreases.

Example: The data given below is about the number of people who got corona in the year 2020 in India between February to July-2020. Construct line graph for this data.

Month	Number of Corona Patients
Feb	3
Mar	48
Apr	4777
May	78057
June	216872
July	1118107

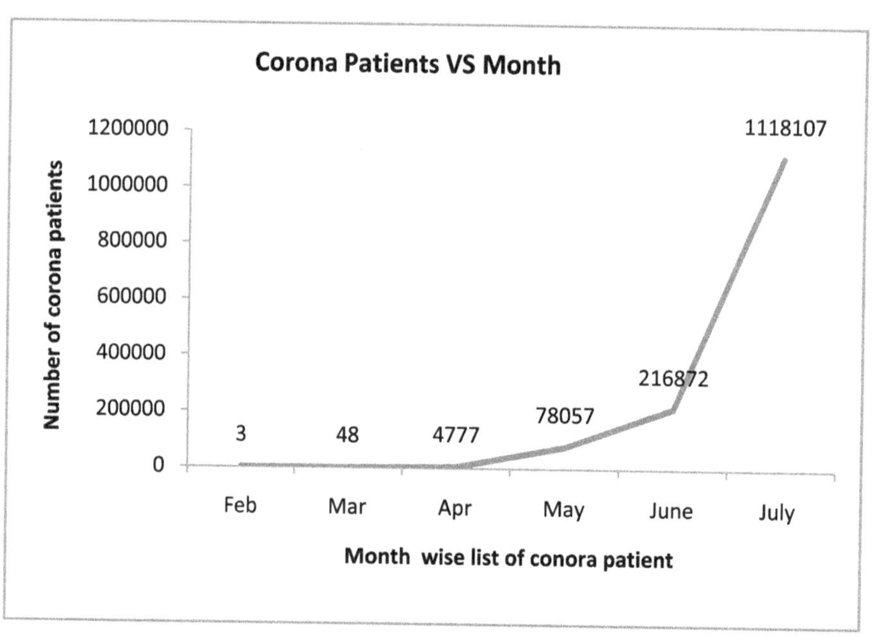

Semilog-graph

This is simply a graph paper which has one linear axis and one log axis. It is used in the case where the data range on one axis is extremely large and/or does not follow a linear progression or the values increase exponentially.

In general to construct graph we use natural scale in which equal distances represent equal absolute magnitude on both of the axes. But in case of phenomena under study increase or decrease in the value of the variable is very rapid. In such a situation we primarily focus on the study of relative changes rather than the absolute changes. When we encounter these type of problems, semi-logarithmic or logarithmic or ratio scale graph used to highlight or emphasize relative changes.

Semi-log plot is a way of visualizing data that are related according to an exponential relationship. One *axis* is plotted on a *logarithmic* scale. The type of curve which obtained by plotting absolute scale on X-axis and logarithmic values on Y-axis is called as Semi-logarithmic graph.

In epidemiology, this type of graph to show a long series of data and to compare several series. It is the method of choice for plotting rates over time.

Shape of the curve on semi-logarithmic scale and natural Scale:

1. The values of data under study is increasing by a constant amount (difference between different interval of time is constant) will give a straight line rising upward when the data is plotted on natural scale, but when same data is plotted on semi-logarithmic scale graph, we will get an upward rising curve. The slope of the curve will be steadily decreasing. That indicates that the decreasing rate is very steady. The curve is concave to the base.

Example **1:** The concentration of drug, which is measured as a function of time is as listed below. Construct the graph on natural scale and also semi-logarithmic scale graph

Time (Weeks)	Concentration	Log (Concentration)
0	0	0
2	10	1
4	20	1.30
6	30	1.48
8	40	1.60
10	50	1.70

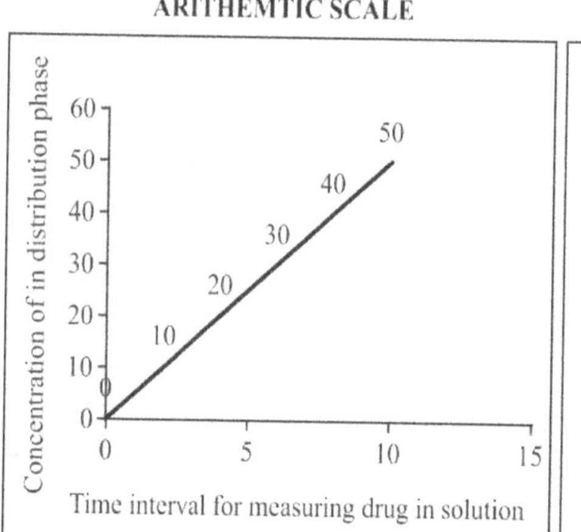

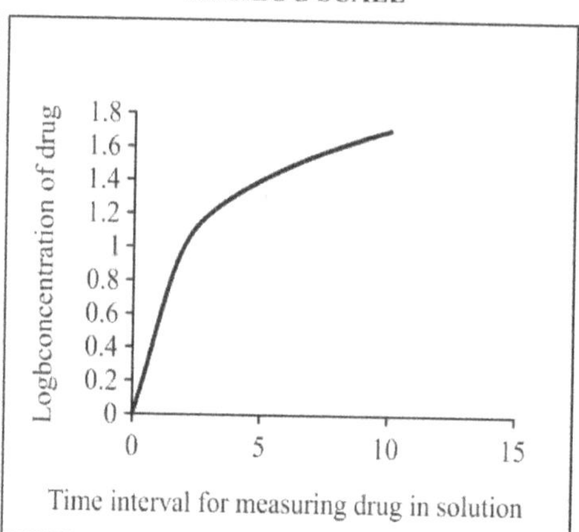

2. The values of data under study is increasing by a constant rate (the ratio between the phenomenon under study at different interval of time is constant) will give a curve convex to the base when data plotted on natural scale and the slope of the curve will be steadily increasing. The same data when they are plotted on semi-logarithmic scale graph, we will get an upward rising straight line.

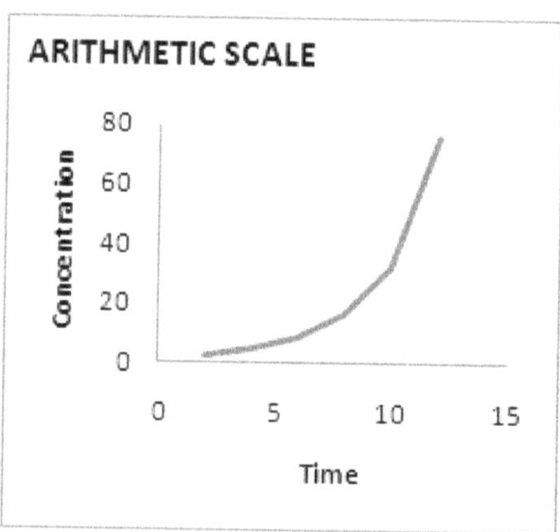

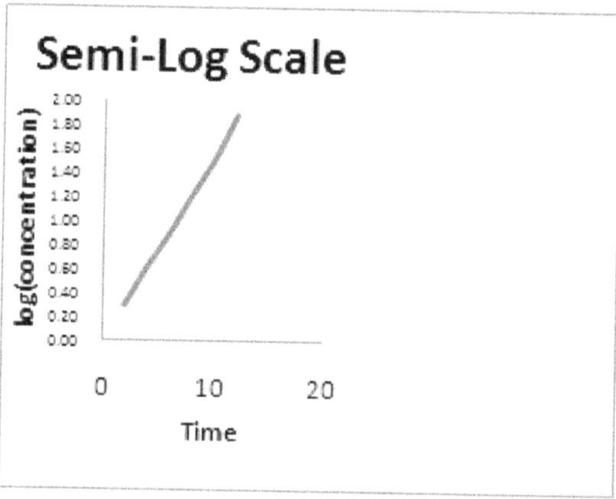

3. The values of data under study is decreasing by a constant amount (difference between different interval of time is constant) will give a straight line falling downward when the data is plotted on natural scale, but when same data are plotted on semi-logarithmic scale graph, we will get an downward falling curve to the right. The slope of the curve will be steadily increasing.

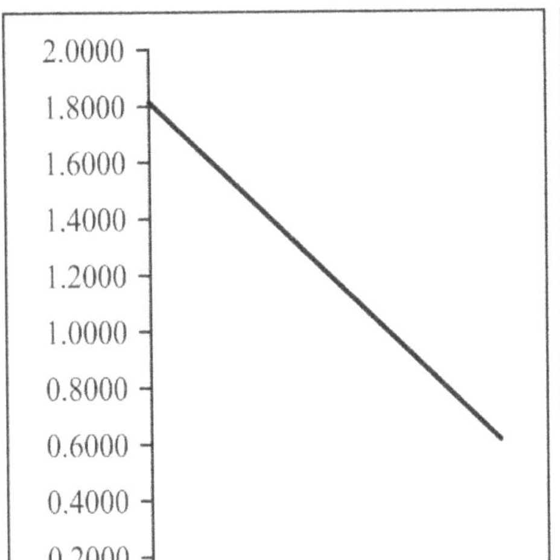

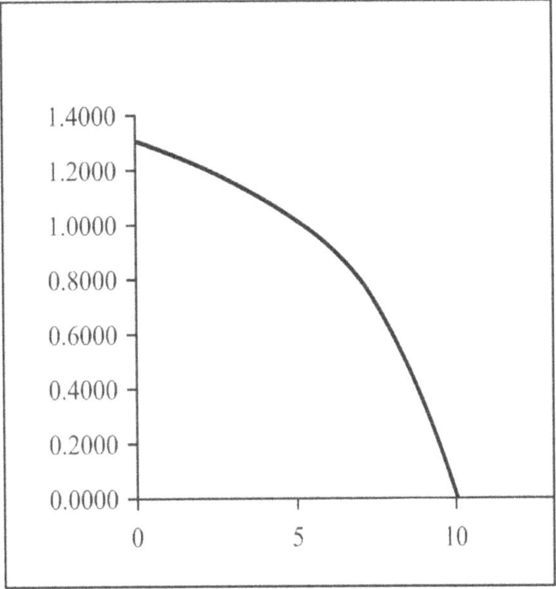

4. The values of data under study is decreasing by a constant rate (the ratio between the phenomenon under study at different interval of time is constant) will give a curve moving downwards with a declining slope when data are plotted on natural scale, but when same data are plotted on semi-logarithmic scale graph, we will get a straight line moving downward.

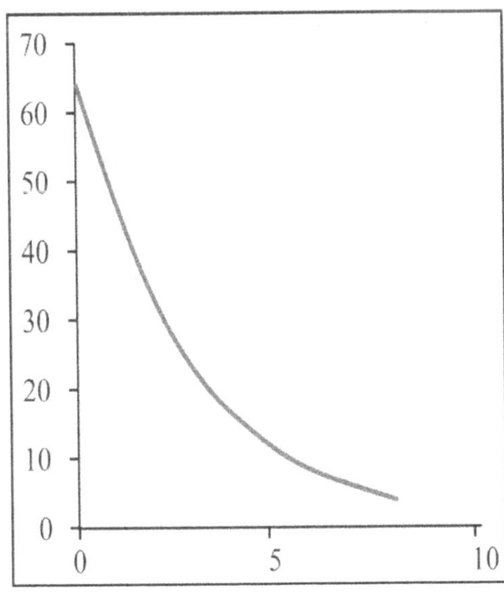

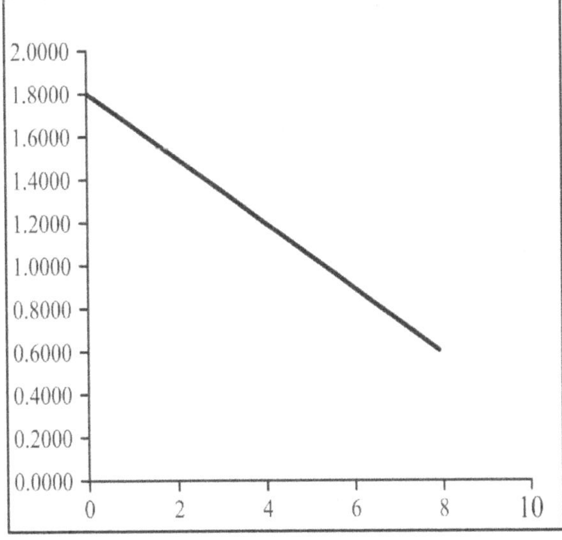

The general format of semi-log graph sheet

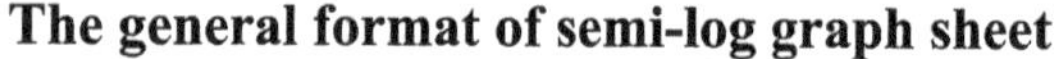

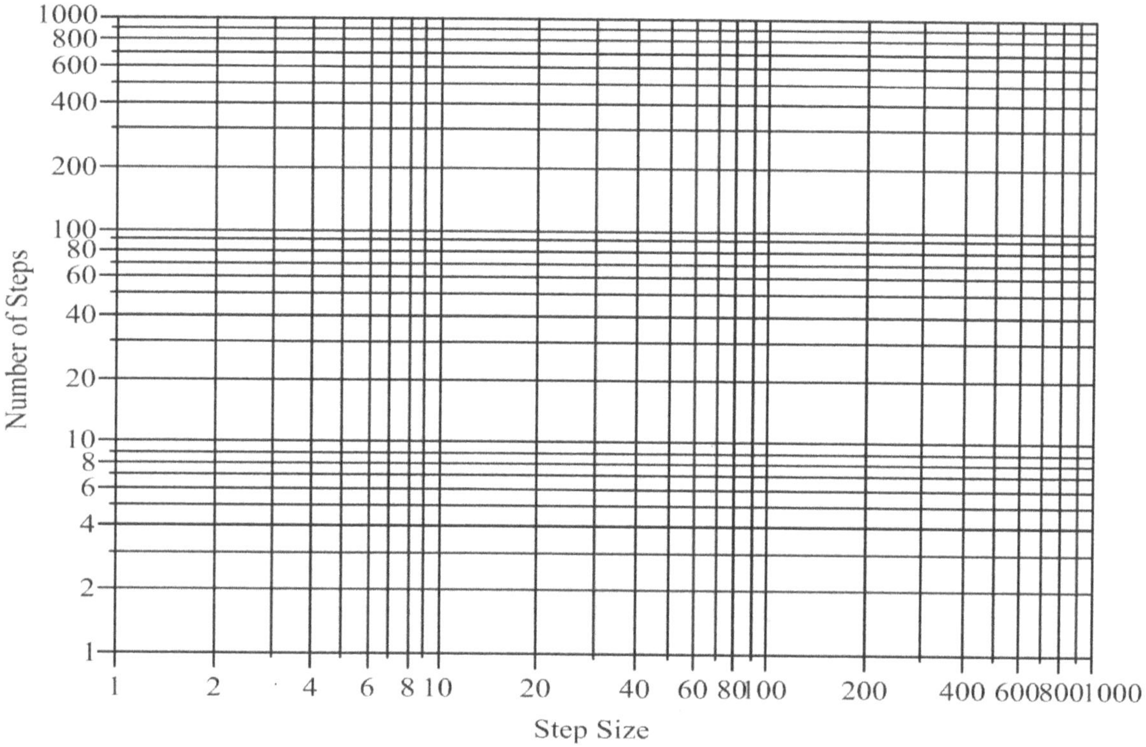

Interpretation of Semi-logarithmic or Ratio Curves

1. If the curve is rising upwards, the rate of growth of phenomenon under study is increasing positively and if curve falls downward that indicates rate of growth phenomenon is decreasing
2. If the curve is nearly a straight line which is moving upward, indicates the rate of change of phenomenon under study is more or less constant. Similarly , if the curve is nearly a straight line and moving downward indicates that the rate of change of phenomenon is decreasing at a uniform rate.
3. If the curve rises (falls) steeply at one point of time, than any another point of time, indicates that there is a rapid rate of increase or decrease at that point of time than any other point of time
4. If two curves of different data on the same semi-logarithmic graph are parallel to each other, then they represent equal percentage of change between both the phenomenon under study.
5. If the first is steeper than the second curve on the same ratio chart, that indicates, the changing rate first is faster than the second

Example: A 3 year old, 15 kg patient was brought in for surgery and was given a 100 mcg/kg by bolus injection of a muscle relaxant. The plasma concentrations were measured post injection and noted in the table below. Construct a semi-log graph

Time (h)	Plasma Conc. (mcg/L)
0.5	100
1	85
3	57
5	37
7	22

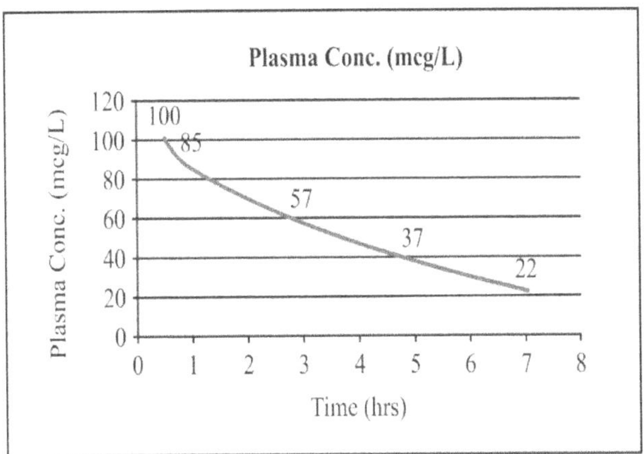

Semi-log Plot of Plasma-level versus time for a two-compartment IV bolus models
Plot on Natural scale

Time	Cp (mg/L)
0.5	100
1	85
3	57
5	37
7	22

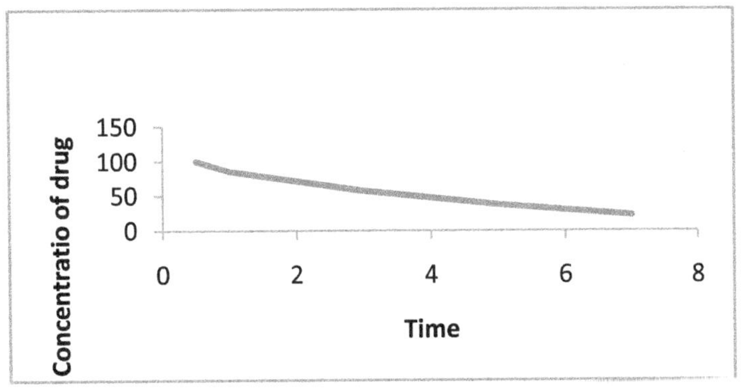

Plot on Semi-log scale Graph

Time	log(Cp)
0.5	2
1	1.93
3	1.76
5	1.57
7	1.34

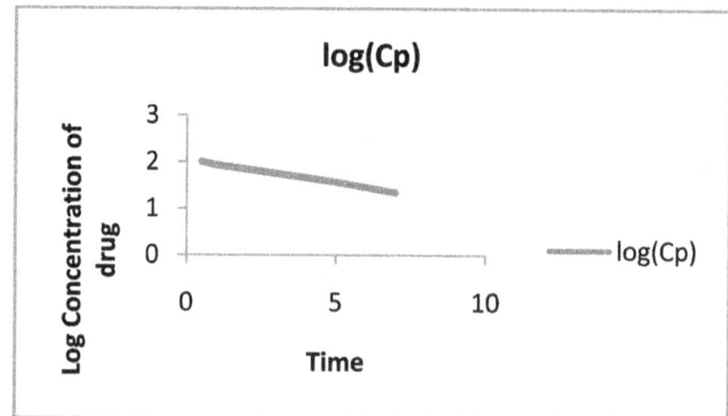

Scatter Diagram Method

Scatter diagram is one of the simplest ways to present data in the form diagram and it will be helpful for ascertaining the correlation between two variables. Suppose there are n-pair of values $(x_1, y_1), (x_2, y_2)$………..(x_n, y_n) of two variables X and Y. This graph will give a rough idea about the relationship between two variables.

1. If the point are very dense, then investigator can conclude that fairly a good amount of correlation exists between two variables
2. The correlation between two variables is said to be positive, if there is an upward trend rising from left hand corner and going upward to the upper right handed corner, otherwise the correlation is said to be negative when the point moves from upper left hand corner to the lower right handed corner.
3. If all the point lie on a line (may be +ve or –ve) then the correlation between them is perfect.
4. If the points lie in a circle or in the form of parabola, this indicates the absence of correlation.

Example: The data given in the table shows the relationship between age and Bilirubin level in each patient. Construct curve and scattered graph

Age X	71	69	80	60	63	49	51	49	52	45
Bilirubin (mg/dl)	11	12.3	14	9.1	7.8	6.5	9	7.5	9	7

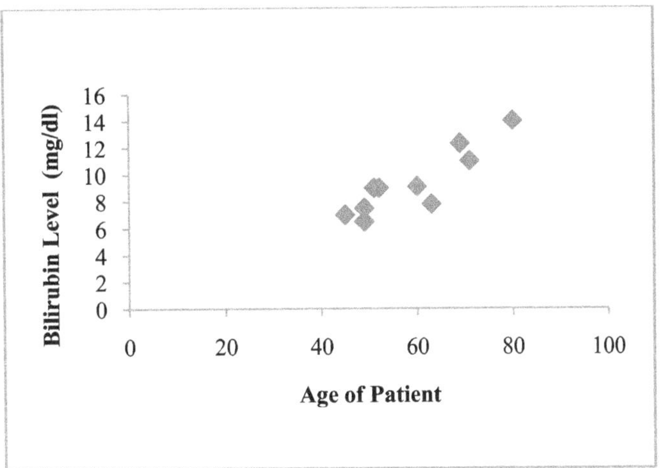

Example: The data given in the table shows the relationship between sugar consumption and dental caries of ten places of state (Mean DMFT). Construct scattered diagram.

SL No	Sugar Consumption	Mean DMFT
01	35.50	2.2
02	13	1.8
03	34.67	3.5
04	35.20	1.8
05	34.76	1.2
06	2.88	3.5
07	46.93	6.5
08	36.50	3.6
09	21.30	6.2
10	25.56	4.6

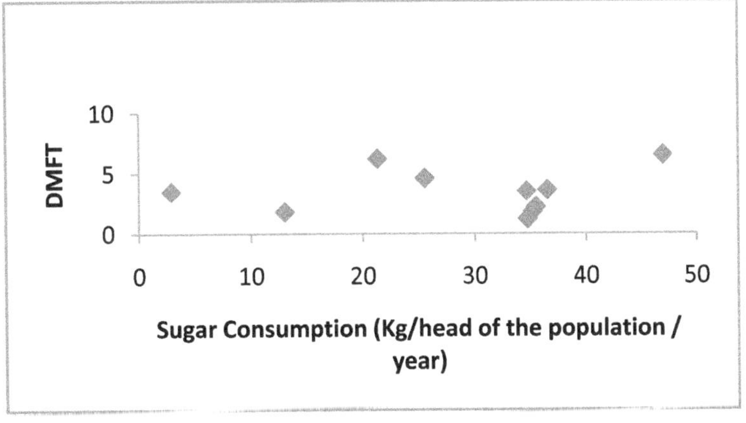

Stem-and-Leaf Diagrams

A stem-and-leaf diagram is a graphical representation in which the data points are grouped in such a way that we can see the shape of the distribution while retaining the individual values of the data points. It is more useful for small data.

A stem-and-leaf diagram consists of a series of rows of numbers. The number used to label a row is called as a stem and other numbers in the row are called as leaves.

Example: The age of 27 patients who have chosen for a pilot study is as listed below. Construct stem-and-leaf diagram for the same data.

SLNO	1	2	3	4	5	6	7	8	9	10	11	12	13	14	15	16	17	18
AGE	20	23	18	29	35	37	29	41	45	50	53	55	60	48	39	47	58	60

	Stems	Leafs			
1	1	8			
2	2	0	3	9	9
3	3	5	7	9	
4	4	1	5	7	8
5	5	0	3	5	8
6	6	0	0		

CHAPTER 11

Clinical Trial

Clinical trials can be considered as a key research tool to enhance the medical knowledge and focus on patient care. Clinical research is done only if doctors do not know whether a new methodology works well on subjects and one can assess the safety, and finally come to the conclusion of which treatment or strategies work best for certain illnesses or group of people.

Clinical trials are very important in discovering new treatments for diseases, as well as for the best way to detect, diagnose, and reduce the chance of developing the disease. Clinical trials can help researchers to know which treatment works well and which one doesn't work in humans, the same cannot be learned through animal trials in the laboratory. Clinical trials also help doctors to decide the extent of the side effects of a new treatment that is acceptable when compared with the potential benefits. Millions of people have benefitted because other people before them chose to participate in a trial that resulted in a new, more effective treatment. Only in rare cases, patient volunteers have been hurt by the treatment or procedure on a clinical trial.

These studies may also assess how effective a medical approach is for specific conditions or groups of people. Overall, they add to the medical knowledge and provide useful information or data to assist in health care decision-making.

Whenever clinical trials are conducted, the investigators should ensure the safety of the participant or subjects during the clinical trial and the trials always start with small groups and examined for the side effects of the treatment during the trail. This is because a technique which was successful in a laboratory when performed on animals may not be safe or effective for human being.

The working procedure of a clinical trial use the method of comparison of groups. The main purpose of comparison is to decide the medical strategies and treatments. Results can be analyzed by comparing the outcome of different groups and one can draw the inference about which group result is more significant. The result of one group may be more significant than the result of other group, because one group receives the existing treatment and the other group will receive the new treatment.

Clinical trials on humans are conducted in the final stages of a long, systematic, and thorough research process. The process often begins in a laboratory, where new concepts are developed and tested. Testing on animals enables scientists to see how the approach affects a living body. Finally, human testing is carried out in small and then in larger groups.

Purpose of Clinical Trials

The purpose of clinical trial is to

1. **Evaluate one or more treatment interventions** for a disease, syndrome or condition, such as drugs, medical devices, or approaches to surgery or therapies
2. **Assess ways to prevent a disease or condition**, for example, through medicines, vaccines, and lifestyle changes
3. **Evaluate one or more diagnosis interventions** that might identify or diagnose a particular disease or condition of subject.
4. **Examine identification methods** for recognizing a condition or risk factors for that condition a patient or subject who has been selected for study
5. **Explore supportive care procedures** to improve the comfort and quality of life of people with chronic diseases like diabetic, asthma etc

Avoiding Bias

Maximum care has to be taken by researchers to avoid bias for allocating the subjects for clinical trials. Bias refers to human choices or other factors that are not related to the protocol but which may affect the results of the trial. The important steps which can avoid bias are comparison groups, randomization, and masking.

Comparison Groups

The common procedure which is applied in clinical trial is the comparison of two groups to compare medical strategies and treatments. Results we get after performing trial will show which group shows better outcome. In this case investigator conduct the experiment in ways as mentioned below

1. One group receives an existing treatment for a condition, and the second group receives a new treatment, then the investigator compare which group has produced better result.
2. One group receives a new treatment, and the second group receives a placebo, an inactive product that looks like the test product.

Randomization

Clinical trials with comparison groups often use randomization. Participants are allocated to comparison groups by chance rather than by choice. This means that any differences seen during a trial will be due to the strategy used and not because of pre-existing differences between participants.

Masking or Blinding

Masking or blinding helps to avoid bias by not informing either the participants or the researchers which treatment will be given to or received by the subjects or participants.

Single blind: The blindness is the policy of keeping someone unaware of which treatment has been given. Studies are said to be single blind, if the subject will be not aware which treatment he or she has received or administered.

Double blind: Intervention studies are double blind if both the doctor, nurse or whoever is going to assess the outcomes (response from subjects, any physical measurement, tests carried out in laboratory), and the subject is unaware of the treatment or drug administered. This can avoid observer bias

Sometimes the person usually the statistician who will interpret the results obtained after performing the interventional study or clinical trial, is also kept blind. Then this type of study is called as **triple blind.**

Confounding Factors

A confounder is one of the factor that can distort the true relationship between two or more characteristics.

For example, one could conclude that people who carry a cigarette lighter are more likely to develop lung cancer because carrying a lighter causes lung cancer. Smoking is a confounder in this example.

People who carry a cigarette lighter are more likely to be smokers, and smokers are more likely to develop lung cancer, but some people may carry a lighter for other purposes. Not taking this point into consideration may lead to false conclusions.

Phases of Clinical Trials

A clinical trial will be done on subjects only, when there is good reason to believe that a new drug or vaccine or treatment may improve the health of patients. Before performing the clinical trials, tests and treatments will be assessed in preclinical studies. Preclinical study will be not on human subjects. It assesses the features of a test or treatment. For example, the research may aim to learn to what extent a device is harmful on living tissue and also one learns more about the chemical makeup of a drug.

After preclinical research, tests and treatments go through a series of clinical trials. Clinical trials assess if tests or treatments are safe for subjects and works well in people. Clinical trials have five phases. The phases are described using the example of a new drug treatment.

Phase 0 Trials: Pharmacodynamics and Pharmacokinetics

Phase 0 trials are the first clinical trials done among people. This is an exploratory phase that helps provide clinical information for a new drug at an earlier phase. Here the investigator can learn how the drug is processed in the body and how it affects the body. In these trials, a very small dose of a drug is given to about 10 to 15 people.

Phase 1 Trials: Screening for Safety

Phase 1 trials are conducted with an aim to find the best dose of a new drug with minimum side effects. The drug will be tested in a small group of 15 to 30 patients. Doctors will administer very low doses of the drug to very few number of subjects. Higher doses are given to other patients until side effects become too severe or the desired effect is seen. The drug may help patients, but the purpose of Phase I is to test the safety of the drug. Once the investigator find that drug is safe enough, then it can be tested in a phase II clinical trial.

Phase 2 Trials: Establishing Effectiveness

Phase 2 trials further it is going to assess effectiveness and safety if a drug works well. The drug is often tested among patients or subjects with a specific type of disease like cancer, HIV etc. Phase II trials are done in larger groups of patients compared to Phase I trials. This study may include any number between 36 and 300 participants or subjects by collecting preliminary data on whether the drug works in people with a certain disease or condition

Often, new combination of drugs are tested. Patients are closely watched to see how the drug works. However, the new drug is rarely compared to the current (standard-of-care) drug that is used or with Placebo. If a drug is found to works well, then it can be tested in a phase III clinical trial.

Phase 3 Trials: Final Confirmation of Safety and Effectiveness

Phase III trials compare a new drug to the standard-of-care drug. These trials assess the side effects of each drug and which drug works better. Phase III trials enroll 100 or more patients.

To perform this trial investigator will go for randomization. Here patients are put into a treatment group, called trial arms, by chance. The randomization process is required to make sure that the people in all trial arms are alike. This allows the investigator or researchers to know that the results of the clinical trial are due to the treatment and not because of differences in groups. A computer program will be used randomly to assign people to the trial group or arms.

There can be more than two treatment groups in phase III trials. The control group gets the standard-of-care treatment. The other groups get a new treatment. Neither you nor your doctor can choose your group. In case of Phase 3 no one will know which group they are allocated, until the trial is over.

Every patient in a phase III study is watched closely. The study will be stopped early if the side effects of the new drug are too severe or if one group has much better results. Phase III clinical trials are often needed before the FDA approves the use of a new drug for the general public.

Phase 4 Trials: Studies during Sales

Phase 4 trials test new drugs approved by the FDA for marketing. The drug will be tested in several hundreds or thousands of patients or subjects. This allows the researchers to know the short–term and long-term side effects and safety of drug. For instance, some rare side effects may only be found in large groups of people. Doctors can also learn and analyze more about how well the drug works and if it is helpful when used with other treatments.

They are designed to include over 1000 patients and comprehensive experience in evaluating the safety and effectiveness of the new medicine in a larger group and subpopulations of patients, comparison and combination with other available treatments and evaluation of long-term side effects of the drug, detection of less common adverse events, cost-effectiveness of drug therapy compared with other traditional and new therapies.

Safety Report

After the FDA approves a drug, the post-marketing stage begins. The sponsorer, usually the manufacturer, submits periodic safety updates to the FDA.

References

1. Charles S. Eby, Prothrombotic states in ischemic stroke, Seminars in Cerebrovascular Diseases and Stroke, Volume 2, Issue 2, June 2002, Pages 90-101

2. P. G. Anastasiadis, P. G. Skaphida, N. G. Koutlaki, G. Ch. Galazios, P. N. Liberis, Epidemiologic aspects of endometrial cancer in Thrace, Greece, International Journal of Gynecology & Obstetrics, Volume 66, Issue 3, 1 September 1999, Pages 263-272

3. M Lejoyeux, M Mc Loughlin, J Adès, Epidemiology of behavioral dependence: literature review and results of original studies , European Psychiatry, Volume 15, Issue 2, March 2000, Pages 129-134

4. Kornelija Mise, Anteo Bradaric, Dragan Arar, Andrija Svilicic, Roko Martinic, P-93 Retrospective study: Epidemiological and histological differences in lung cancer 1980–2001 in South Croatia, Lung Cancer,Volume 41, Supplement 2, August 2003, Page S114

5. C. K. Connolly, M. Mamun, S. M. Alcock, R. J. Prescott, The Darlington and North allerton, prospective asthma study: best function predicts mortality during the first 10 years, Respiratory Medicine, Volume 92, Issue 11, November 1998, Pages 1274-1280

6. Pelayo Correa, William Haenszel. The Epidemiology of Large-Bowel Cancer , Advances in Cancer Research, Volume 26, 1978, Pages 1-141

7. M. Joachim, M. Tuizer, S. Araidy, I. Abu El-Naaj, Pediatric maxillofacial trauma: epidemilogic study between the years 2012–2015 in Israeli medical center, International Journal of Oral and Maxillofacial Surgery, Volume 48, Supplement 1, May 2019, Page 40

8. Li-Zhen Chen, Xinru Yuan, Yuanchao Zhang, Shu Zhang, Gao-Xia Wei, Brain Functional Specialization Is Enhanced Among Tai *Chi* Chuan Practitioners, Archives of Physical Medicine and Rehabilitation, Volume 101, Issue 7, July 2020, Pages 1176-1182

9. Anne-Laure Boulesteix, Carolin Strobl, Maximally selected *Chi-squared* statistics and non-monotonic associations: An exact approach based on two cut points, Computational Statistics & Data Analysis, Volume 51, Issue 12, 15 August 2007, Pages 6295-6306.

10. JEFFREY A. GLINER, GEORGE A. MORGAN, ROBERT J. HARMON, The Chi-Square Test and Accompanying Effect Size Indices, Journal of the American Academy of Child & Adolescent Psychiatry, Volume 41, Issue 12, December 2002, Pages 1510-1512

11. Cristina Godoy, Paula Peremiquel-Trillas, Cristina Andrés, Laura Gimferrer, Andrés Antón A molecular epidemiological study of human parainfluenza virus type 3 at a tertiary university hospital during 2013–2015 in Catalonia, Spain, Diagnostic Microbiology and Infectious Disease ,Volume 86, Issue 2, October 2016, Pages 153-159

12. The role of pesticide exposure in the genesis of Parkinson's disease: Epidemiological studies and experimental data, Toxicology, Volume 307, 10 May 2013, Pages 24-34,

13. G. Chartier, D. Cawthorpe, From 'Big 4' to 'Big 5': A review and epidemiological study on the relationship between psychiatric disorders and World Health Organization preventable diseases, European Psychiatry, Volume 41, Supplement, April 2017, Page S489

14. D. A. M. Twisk, Martine Reurings, An epidemiological study of the risk of cycling in the dark: The role of visual perception, conspicuity and alcohol use, Accident Analysis & Prevention, Volume 60, November 2013, Pages 134-140

15. Ying Lian, Qun Yuan, Gangpu Wang, Fang Tang, Association between sleep quality and metabolic syndrome: A systematic review and meta-analysis, Psychiatry Research Volume 274, April 2019, Pages 66-74

16. Juliette Raffort, Réda Hassen-Khodja, Elixène Jean-Baptiste, Fabien Lareyre, Relationship between metformin and abdominal aortic aneurysm, Journal of Vascular Surgery, Volume 71, Issue 3, March 2020, Pages 1056-1062

17. J. A. Olmos, R. Higa, H. Ríos, L. O. Soifer, E. Varela, Association between subjects with dyspeptic sumptoms and Helicobacter pylori infection: Epidemilogic Study conducted at 16 centers in Argentina, Gastroenterology, Volume 114, Supplement 1, 15 April 1998, Page A248

18. Ji Zeng, Chan Lu, Qihong Deng, Prenatal exposure to diurnal temperature variation and early childhood pneumonia, Journal of Thermal Biology, Volume 65, April 2017, Pages 105-112

19. Serap Hasturk, Ismail Hanta, Sedat Kuleci, Serap Duru P-97 No change the relationship of lung cancer and smoking behavior for Turkey: Based on the hospital population in the South of Turkey, Lung Cancer, Volume 41, Supplement 2, August 2003, Page S115

20. I. Bibou-Nakou, A. Markos, S. Padeliadu, P. Chatzilampou, S. Ververidou Multi-informant evaluation of students' psychosocial status through SDQ in a national Greek sample, Children and Youth Services Review, Volume 96, January 2019, Pages 47-54

21. Grazyna Jasienska, Anna Ziomkiewicz, Maciej Górkiewicz, Andrzej Pająk, Body mass, depressive symptoms and menopausal status: An examination of the "Jolly Fat" hypothesis, Women's Health Issues, Volume 15, Issue 3, May–June 2005, Pages 145-151

22. E. C. Hedberg, Stephanie Ayers, The power of a *paired t-test* with a covariate, Social Science Research, Volume 50, March 2015, Pages 277-291

23. Charles J. Kowalski, Emet D. Schneiderman, Stephen M. Willis, PC program implementing an alternative to the paired *t*-test which adjusts for regression to the mean, International Journal of Bio-Medical Computing, Volume 37, Issue 3, November–December 1994, Pages 189-194

24. Xumin Ni, Chendi Zhu, Qing Li, Hui Jiang, Weimin Li, Epidemiology characteristics of the clonal complexes of *Mycobacterium tuberculosis* Lineage 4 in China, Infection, Genetics and Evolution, Volume 84, October 2020, 104363

25. Chenzhi Hou, Zhendong Hua, Peng Xu, Hui Xu, Bin Di, Estimating the prevalence of hepatitis B by wastewater-based epidemiology in 19 cities in China, Science of The Total Environment, Volume 740, 20 October 2020, 139696

26. Aiko Tanaka,Kate Hamilton,Glenn M. Eastwood, Daryl Jones, Rinaldo Bellomo, The epidemiology of overfeeding in mechanically ventilated intensive care patients, Clinical Nutrition ESPEN, Volume 36, April 2020, Pages 139-145

27. Candice Y. Johnson, Penelope P. Howards, Matthew J. Strickland, D. Kim Waller, The National Birth Defects Prevention *Study Multiple* bias analysis using *logistic regression*: an example from the National Birth Defects Prevention *Study*, Annals of Epidemiology, Volume 28, Issue 8, August 2018, Pages 510-514

28. G. Tripepi, K. J. Jager, F. W. Dekker, C. Zoccali, Linear and *logistic regression* analysis, Kidney International, Volume 73, Issue 7, 1 April 2008, Pages 806-810

29. Saverio Caini, Doménica de Mora, Maritza Olmedo, Denisses Portugal, Alfredo Bruno, The *epidemiology* and severity of respiratory viral infections in a tropical country: Ecuador, 2009–2016,Journal of Infection and Public Health, Volume 12, Issue 3, May–June 2019, Pages 357-363

30.S. Blagden V. Watts, N. Q. Verlander, M. Pegorie, Invasive group A streptococcal infections in North West England: epidemiology, risk factors and fatal infection, Volume 186, September 2020, Pages 63-70

31. Sharareh Eskandarieh, Saharnaz Nedjat, Ibrahim Abdollahpour, Abdorreza Naser, Moghadasi, Mohammad Ali Sahraian, Comparing epidemiology and baseline characteristic of multiple sclerosis and neuromyelitis optica: A case-control study. Multiple Sclerosis and Related Disorders, Volume 12, February 2017, Pages 39-43

32. Jacob C. Jentzer, Thomas Breen, Mandeep Sidhu, Gregory W. Barsness, Kianoush Kashani,Epidemiology and outcomes of acute kidney injury in cardiac intensive care unit patients, Journal of Critical Care, Volume 60, December 2020, Pages 127-134

33. Chun-Pin Chang, Shen-Chih Chang, Shu-Chun Chuang, Julien Berthiller, Yuan-Chin Amy Lee, Age at start of using tobacco on the risk of head and neck cancer: Pooled analysis in the International Head and Neck, Cancer Epidemiology, Volume 63, December 2019, 101615 (INHANCE).

34. Xiaowei Chen,Zhaofei Pang, Yu Wang, Fenglong Bie, Jiajun Du, The role of surgery for atypical bronchopulmonary carcinoid tumor: Development and validation of a model based on Surveillance, Epidemiology, and End Results (SEER) database, Lung Cancer, Volume 139, January 2020, Pages 94-102

35. H. A. Lee, N. Son, W. K. Lee, Association between dietary patterns derived by reduced rank *regression* and incident diabetes: From the korean genome *epidemiology study* Clinical Nutrition September 2018, Clinical Nutrition, Volume 37, Supplement 1, September 2018, Pages S97-S98.

36. David Polo, Marcos Quintela-Baluja, Alexander Corbishley, Davey L. Jones, Jesús L., Romalde, Making waves: Wastewater-based *epidemiology* for COVID-19 – approaches and challenges for surveillance and prediction, Water Research, Volume 186, 1 November 2020, 116404

37. Ellen Moscoe, Jacob Bor, Till Bärnighausen, The global epidemiology of anabolic-androgenic steroid use: a meta-analysis and meta-regression analysis, Volume 24, Issue 5, May 2014, Pages 383-398

38. Roger J. Marshall, The use of classification and regression trees in clinical epidemiology Journal of Clinical Epidemiology, Volume 54, Issue 6, June 2001, Pages 603-609

39. Li Fan, Jing Zhao, Wen Li, the extension of 2-in-1 adaptive phase 2/3 designs and its application in oncology clinical trials, Contemporary Clinical Trials, Volume 98, November 2020, 106148

39. Rachael Liu, Jianchang Lin, Pin Li, Design considerations for phase I/II dose finding clinical trials in Immuno-oncology and cell therapy, Contemporary Clinical Trials, Volume 96, September 2020, 106083

40. Katharina Hees, Meinhard Kieser, Blinded sample size recalculation in clinical trials incorporating historical data, Contemporary Clinical Trials, Volume 63, December 2017, Pages 2-7

41. Kung-Jong Lui, Chii-Dean Lin, Sample size determination for cluster randomization phase II trials of dichotomous data, Statistical Methodology, Volume 5, Issue 5, September 2008, Pages 474-485

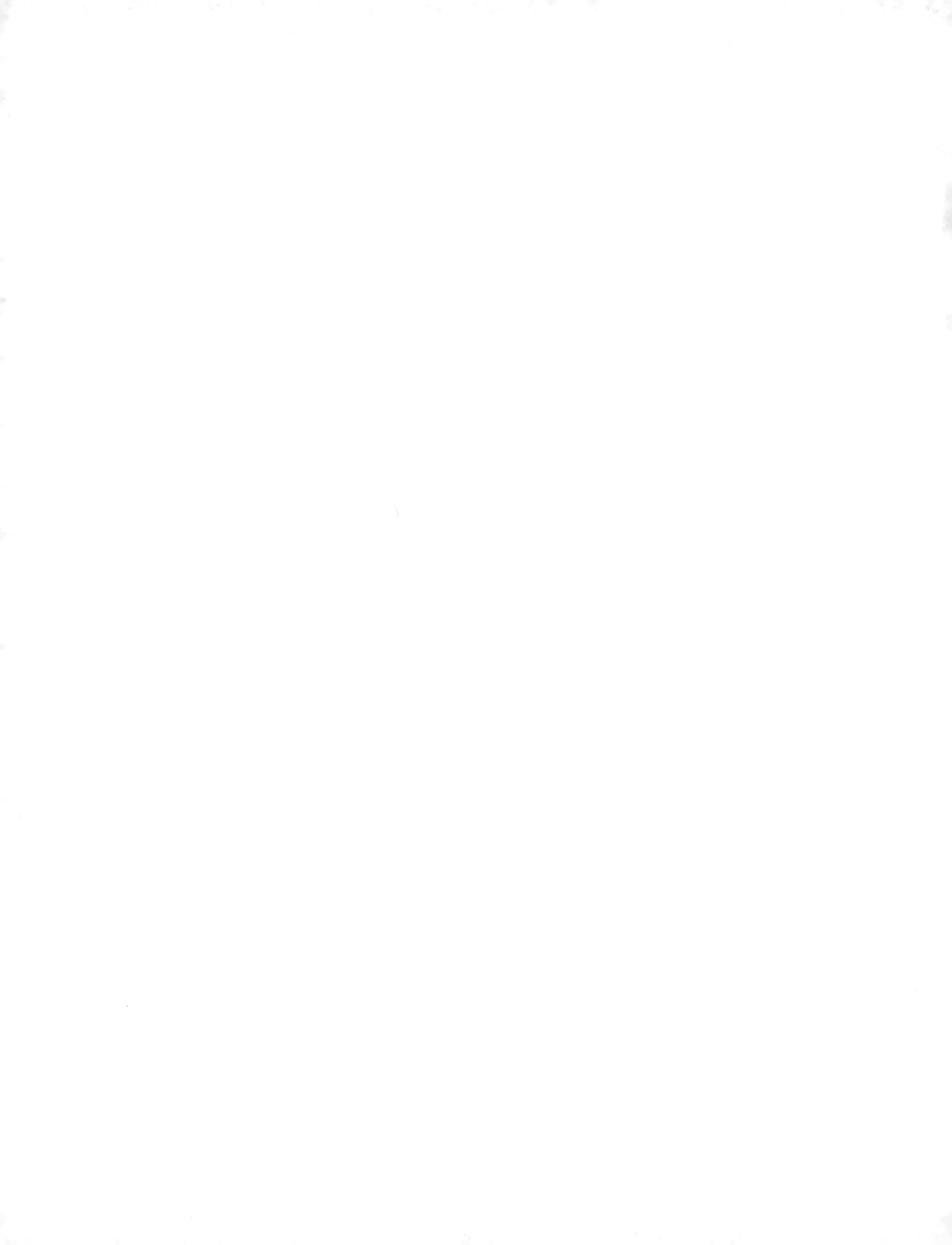